# The distal radial approach in interventional cardiology

Mourad BOUKHELOUA
Mohamed BERREHAL

**Mourad BOUKHELOUA**
**Mohamed BERREHAL**

# The distal radial approach in interventional cardiology

**ScienciaScripts**

**Imprint**

Any brand names and product names mentioned in this book are subject to trademark, brand or patent protection and are trademarks or registered trademarks of their respective holders. The use of brand names, product names, common names, trade names, product descriptions etc. even without a particular marking in this work is in no way to be construed to mean that such names may be regarded as unrestricted in respect of trademark and brand protection legislation and could thus be used by anyone.

Cover image: www.ingimage.com

This book is a translation from the original published under ISBN 978-620-3-46163-3.

Publisher:
Sciencia Scripts
is a trademark of
Dodo Books Indian Ocean Ltd. and OmniScriptum S.R.L publishing group

120 High Road, East Finchley, London, N2 9ED, United Kingdom
Str. Armeneasca 28/1, office 1, Chisinau MD-2012, Republic of Moldova, Europe
Printed at: see last page
**ISBN: 978-620-6-25174-3**

# THE DISTAL RADIAL APPROACH IN INTERVENTIONAL CARDIOLOGY
## MOURAD BOUKHELOUA MOHAMED BERREHAL

*2023*

# TABLE OF CONTENTS

# PREFACE

The distal radial approach in interventional cardiology is an innovative and promising technique that uses an artery more superficial than the proximal radial artery primarily in coronary angiography and coronary angioplasty procedures, and perhaps in other types of procedure in the future. This technique offers several advantages over the conventional or femoral approach, including reduced risk of bleeding, vascular complications and pain, and essentially reduced risk of radial artery occlusion, as well as improved patient comfort and quality of life.However, this approach requires a longer learning curve and mastery of specific catheterization techniques, as it can sometimes be limited by anatomical difficulties or individual variations. The distal radial approach is an attractive option in interventional cardiology for eligible patients, which can improve clinical outcomes and patient satisfaction. Its use is set to become more widespread in interventional cardiology centers, pending its inclusion in recommendations to make it a reference technique.

**INTRODUCTION**

The development of interventional cardiology has enabled physicians to gain a better understanding of the pathophysiological mechanisms of ischemic heart disease, and above all to provide patients with high-quality care, including revascularization of almost all coronary stenoses, including chronic total occlusions (CTO).Interventional cardiology is not confined to coronary artery disease, but has extended its scope to congenital heart disease and peripheral vascular disorders. The same techniques have also been used in radiology and neurology for various types of pathology.What these so-called interventional procedures have in common, apart from being very simple and comfortable for the patient, is that they all require a peripheral vascular access point. Traditionally, puncture of the femoral artery has been the gold standard, due to its ease of use and the fact that it can accept bulky material.Over the past 30 years, the radial approach has established itself as the preferred route, due to the reduction in access-site complications (hematomas, arteriovenous fistulas) a n d improved patient comfort thanks to early mobilization[1]. Compared with trans femoral access (TFA), trans radial access (TRA) has a similar success rate and is associated with a significantly lower risk of all-cause mortality and major adverse cardiovascular events (MACE)[2]. This advantage exists even in patients with acute coronary syndrome (ACS)[3]. Its popularity and low level of complications have made it the recommended first-line approach (class I) in the recommendations of the European[4] and American Societies of Cardiology[5].

More recently, distal radial access (DRA) has emerged as an alternative to conventional radial access (CRA), minimizing the risk of limb ischemia, putting patient and physician in a more comfortable position and achieving more effective hemostasis in less time.In the light of recent data in the literature, we propose in this booklet to review when and how this innovative technique first appeared, what its advantages and disadvantages are, and what tangible evidence supports this alternative of choice to the radial approach.

# HISTORY OF THE TRANSRADIAL DISTAL

Transradial access was first evaluated in a study in 1948 by Radner Stig[6], when this approach was shown to be an alternative technique for thoracic aortography, which was then performed by injecting contrast medium via the vein and then imaging after the medium had passed into the arterial system. The result was disappointing, with a 25% failure rate. In this context, Radner described the first procedure, in which the radial artery is stripped and a surgical incision of a few millimeters is made, enabling a probe to be introduced retrograde to the aorta (Fig.1.).

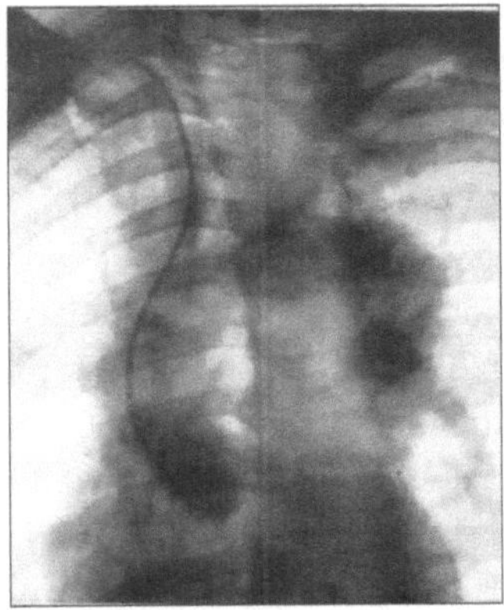

Figure 1. Transradial retrograde aortography [6].

Later, in 1989, Campeau described its use for coronary angiography in a series of 100 patients as an alternative to the brachial approach [7]. Subsequently, the work of Kiemeneij and Laarman demonstrated that transradial access is feasible for a large number of patients. percutaneous coronary intervention with stent implantation in three patients[8]. In the ensuing years, transradial access has established itself as the technique of choice, considerably reducing access-related cardiovascular adverse events compared with the transfemoral route. A 2018 analysis of the Cochrane Database showed that transradial access had fewer access-site complications than transfemoral access (RR 0.36, 95% CI 0.22 to 0.59; 16,112 participants in 24 studies)[9]. The American and European Societies of Cardiology currently recommend transradial access as the preferred approach for all coronary angiography and coronary angioplasty procedures. This complication is rarely symptomatic (especially if the palmar arch is defective), but in its asymptomatic form its incidence varies between 1-30%

according to studies, this variation being essentially due to diagnostic errors[10], [11]. Although most of these occlusions are occult and without ischemic syndrome, they preclude future use of the radial artery, including repeated access for scheduled angioplasty, for example, or the establishment of an arteriovenous fistula in chronic renal failure, etc. Other complications of this approach are summarized in figure 2.

- Non-occlusive lesions of the radial artery: very frequent
- Radial artery spasm: 2-30%.
- Perforation of the radial artery: 0.1-1
- Pseudo aneurysm: 0.1 - 0.44
- Arteriovenous fistulas: < 0.04
- Granuloma at puncture site: 2.8
- Major bleeding at the puncture site: rare

Figure 2: Summary of complications associated with radial access [10].

Furthermore, in cases of tortuosity of the right radial artery, vasospasm or occlusion, or angiography of a left internal mammary bridge, the physician is obliged to choose the left radial artery as the access route. The patient's hand is restricted to a semi-pronation position during the operation, which increases discomfort for the patient. patient. The most awkward situations are those of an obese patient and a short operator, which considerably increases discomfort not only for the patient but also for the operator. As a result, new approaches to puncture are expected, with fewer vascular complications, greater patient comfort and preservation of the traditional radial artery wherever possible.

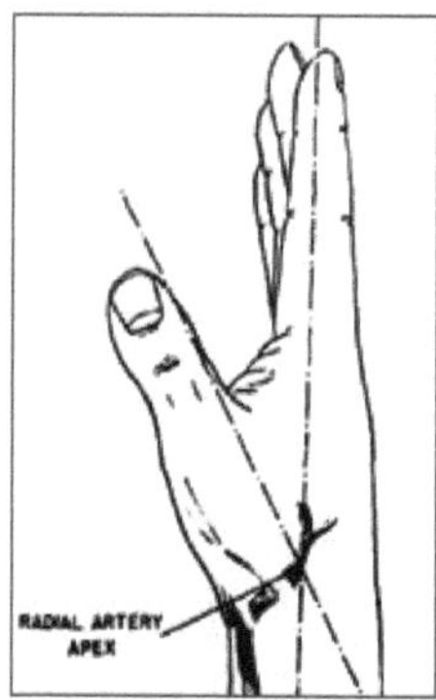

Figure 3: Illustrates the point at which the pulse of the dorsal radial artery is perceptible. [12]

The distal radial approach was first used by anaesthetists as an alternative method of invasive blood pressure measurement[12]. In 1977, Amato described a technique based on puncture of the distal radial artery (Fig.3), as part of the continuous monitoring of blood gases and blood pressure during the perioperative period in cardiac children.He found this approach to be reliable compared with the other approaches used at the time (umbilical, femoral, tibial or temporal...).and that the distal artery remains pulsatile and usable despite iterative punctures of the classic radial and that the pulse has disappeared from the forearm.It wasn't until 2011 that interventional cardiology's interest in the distal radial was revived with the work of Babunashvili and Dundua [13], where this approach was used as a retrograde revascularization approach to the occluded radial artery, with these authors concluding in their publication that:
• In case of radial artery occlusion, the recanalization procedure as a first step is possible and reasonable and the contralateral radial can be preserved for future interventions or as a graft ;
• Recanalization via distal access does not significantly prolong total procedure time or radiation exposure dose;

• This technique can be useful when traditional femoral access is impossible. Subsequently, in 2016, this approach was adapted to coronary procedures with the study by Roghani-Dejkordi et al, who highlighted the feasibility and advantages of the distal approach[14].

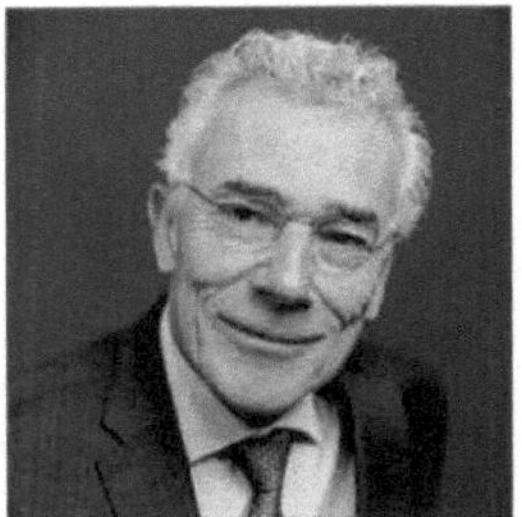

Figure 4: Ferdinand Kiemeneij*, MD, PhD Department of Cardiology, Tergooi Blaricum, Blaricum, the Netherlands


Based on this experience, an initial work published in EuroIntervention in 2017 promoting the distal left approach for coronary procedures was presented by Kiemeneij et al, who shared the experience of 70 patients selected from 118 patients who underwent cardiac catheterization via the distal left radial artery at the level of the anatomical snuffbox, these procedures were performed with 4, 5 and 6 Fr catheters, in stable and acute patients, for simple and complex lesions, and whose puncture methods, procedural data results and complications were Passage through the left hand at the level of the anatomical snuffbox has been proven safe and more comfortable for both the patient and the operator, who is no longer obliged to bend over to reach the left hand[15]. These discoveries gave rise to a rich debate on social networks, highlighting the contribution of social networks to the sharing of scientific experiments. Notably within the @RadialFirst community on Twitter. This was followed by numerous studies comparing the distal radial approach with the conventional radial approach, pioneered by Squeglia et al. al [16] and the study by shunsuke in 2019 comparing the conventional approach with the distal approach. These studies not only demonstrated the feasibility of the distal approach, but also its advantage in terms of radial artery occlusion risk, bleeding risk and compression time, which significantly improved patient comfort.

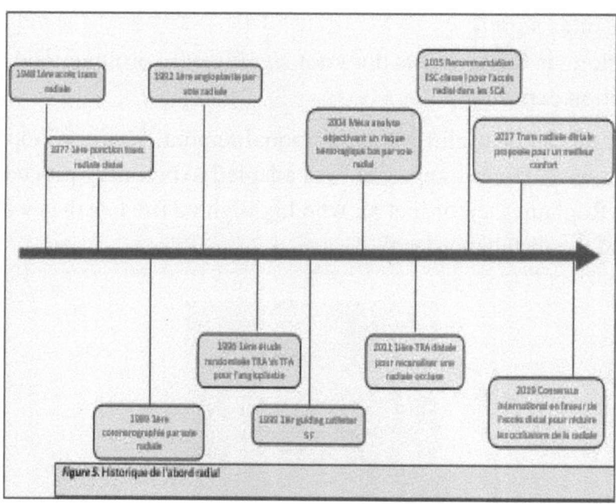

Figure 5: History of the radial approach

More recently, the DiscoTrial trial, an international multicenter study designed to demonstrate the superiority of the distal radial approach compared with a conventional approach. This study demonstrated a clear reduction in the incidence of radial occlusion, a higher rate of repermeabilization after occlusion, shorter hemostasis and a lower risk of bleeding, at the cost of a relatively longer approach time[17]. Figure 5 summarizes the main dates of the radial and distal radial approaches.

# VASCULAR ANATOMY OF THE HAND AND FOREARM

Knowledge and understanding of the vascular anatomy of the hand and arm is essential for safe transradial surgery in general, and distal radial access in particular. This knowledge must include identification of the various arteries and branches, with their luminal diameters, pathways and anatomical variants, as well as the surrounding structures and anatomical compartments in which they are found. We also need to understand the elements of the dual vascularization of the hand by the radial and ulnar arteries.

## I. THE SUBCLAVIAN ARTERY

The arterial supply to the upper limb comes from the subclavian artery, a paired vessel of the thorax. The subclavian arteries are among the largest arteries in the thorax and neck, and are located just below the clavicles. The right and left arteries have different origins The right subclavian artery arises from the brachiocephalic trunk at the same time as the right common carotid artery, and is the first branch of the aortic arch. The left subclavian artery arises directly from the aortic arch, of which it is the third branch, just downstream of the origin of the left common carotid artery.

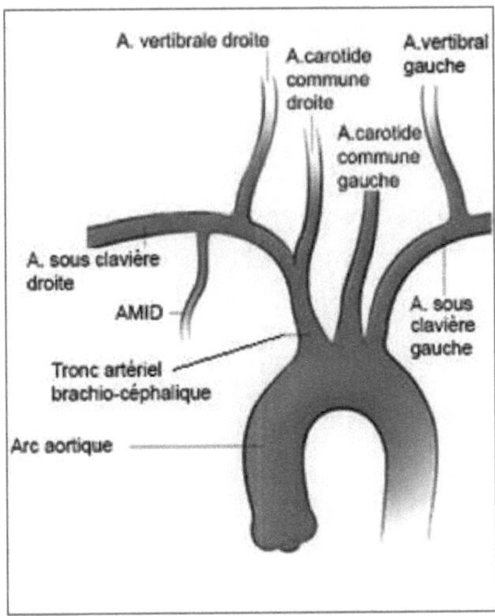


Figure 6: Aorta and supra-aortic trunks

From their origin, the left and right subclavian arteries arch superiorly and laterally towards the axillary region.Along the way, they go through a series of behind the anterior scalene muscles and in front of the middle scalene muscles. Depending on their relationship to the anterior scalene muscles, the subclavian arteries can be divided into three parts:

• **Pre-scalene part**: the part located before the medial border of the anterior scalene muscle.

• **Retro scalene**: the part behind the anterior scalene muscle.

• **Post-scalene part**: part located after the lateral edge of the anterior scalene muscle.

It gives rise to several branches for the head, neck and thorax, as well as scapular branches, before becoming the axillary artery at the lateral edge of the first rib.

## II.THE AXILLARY ARTERY

The axillary artery is a large muscular vessel that crosses the armpit. It supplies blood to the upper limb, as well as parts of the musculocutaneous system of the scapula and upper-lateral thorax. It is a continuation of the subclavian artery, beginning at the outer edge of the first rib and ending at the lower edge of the round tendon, where it is known as the brachial artery[18]. Its direction varies according to the position of the limb; thus, the vessel is almost straight when the arm is directed at right angles to the trunk, concave upwards when the arm is raised above the trunk, and convex upwards and to the side when the arm is extended to the side. At its origin, the artery is very deep, but near its termination, it is superficial, covered only by skin and fascia.

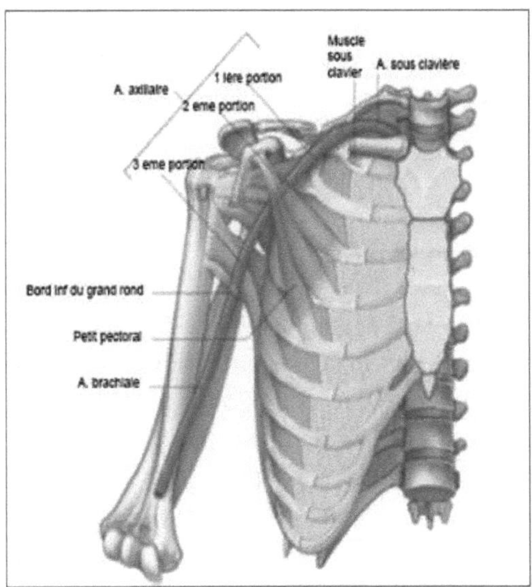


Figure 7. Axillary artery [19]

The vessel is divided into three parts[19] :
• The first portion of the axillary artery is covered anteriorly by the clavicular part of the pectoralis major and the coraco-clavicular fascia, and is crossed by the anterolateral thoracic nerve and the thoracoacromial and cephalic veins. and cephalic veins; posteriorly, the first intercostal space; on its lateral surface, the brachial plexus, from which it is separated by a little loose connective tissue; on its medial, or thoracic, surface, the axillary vein, which overlaps
the artery. Together with the axillary vein and brachial plexus, it is enclosed in a fibrous sheath, the "axillary sheath", which is continuous with the deep cervical fascia.

• The second portion of the axillary artery is covered, anteriorly, by the pectoralis major and minor; posteriorly, there is the posterior cord of the brachial plexus and some loose connective tissue between the artery and the subscapularis; on the medial side, we find the axillary vein, separated from the artery by the medial cord of the brachial plexus and the medial anterior thoracic nerve; on the lateral side, we find the lateral cord of the brachial plexus. brachial plexus. The brachial plexus therefore surrounds the artery on three sides, separating it from direct contact with the vein and adjacent muscles.

• The third portion of the axillary artery extends from the lower edge of the pectoralis minor to the lower edge of the round tendon. Anteriorly, it is covered by the lower part of the pectoralis major above, but only by the integument and fascia below; posteriorly, it is connected to the lower part of the subscapularis and the tendons of the latissimus dorsi and latissimus magnus; on its lateral surface is the coraco brachii, and on its medial or thoracic surface, the axillary vein.

## III. THE BRACHIAL ARTERY

The brachial artery (BA) is the continuation of the main arterial supply in the upper arm, towards the elbow. It begins at the lower edge of the round tendon and, as it descends the It runs the length of the arm, ending about 1 cm below the elbow crease, where it divides into the radial and ulnar arteries[20]. Initially, the brachial artery lies medial to the humerus, but as it moves down the arm, it gradually passes in front of the bone and, at the elbow, it lies midway between its two epicondyles.The artery is superficial throughout, covered at the front by the integument and superficial and deep aponeuroses; the biceps aponeurosis lies in front of it, opposite the elbow. and separates it from the median ulnar vein; the median nerve crosses it from lateral to medial, opposite the insertion of the coraco-brachial. Posteriorly, it is separated from the long head of the triceps brachii by the radial nerve and the deep artery of the arm. It then rests on the medial head of the triceps brachii, then on the insertion of the coraco-brachial and finally on the brachialis. Laterally, it is connected above to the median nerve and the Coraco-brachial, and below to the Biceps brachii, both muscles overlapping the artery to a large extent. Medially, its upper half is connected to the medial antibrachial cutaneous nerve and ulnar nerve, its lower half to the median nerve. The basilic vein lies on its medial side, but is separated from it in the lower arm by the deep fascia.

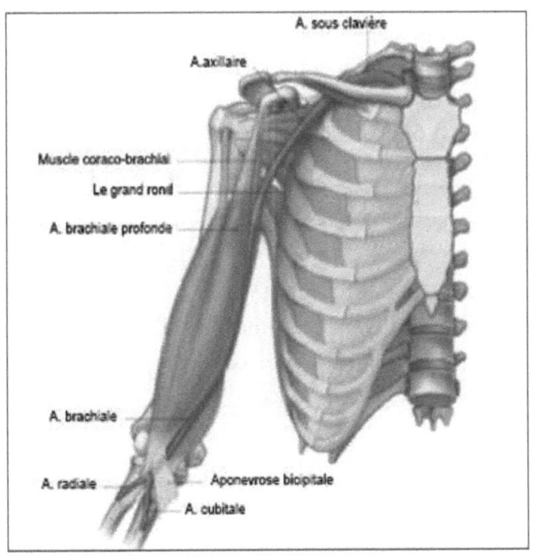



Figure 8. Brachial artery [19]

The artery is accompanied by two satellite veins, which are in close contact with it and are connected at regular intervals by short transverse branches. At the elbow, the brachial artery runs deep into a triangular space known as the anticubital fossa. The base of the triangle points upwards and is represented by a line connecting the two epicondyles of the humerus; the sides are formed by the medial edge of the brachioradialis muscle and the lateral edge of the pronator muscle; the floor is formed by the brachialis and the supinator. This space contains the brachial artery and its accessory veins, the radial and ulnar arteries, the median and radial nerves and the biceps brachii tendon. The brachial artery occupies the middle of the space and divides, opposite the neck of the radius, into the radial (RA) and ulnar (UA) arteries; it is covered, anteriorly, by the integument, the superficial aponeurosis and the median ulnar vein, the latter being separated from the artery by the bicipital aponeurosis. Behind it, the brachial muscle separates it from the elbow joint. The median nerve is close to the medial side of the artery at the top, but is separated at the bottom by the ulnar head of the round pronator muscle. The biceps brachii tendon lies on the lateral side of the artery; the radial nerve is located on the supinator and hidden by the brachioradialis.In some cases, the brachial artery, accompanied by the median nerve, may leave the medial border of the biceps brachii and descend towards the medial epicondyle of the humerus; In this case, it generally passes behind the supracondylar process of the humerus, from which a fibrous arch is most often projected onto the artery; it then passes under or through the substance of the pronator ring muscle, up to the elbow curvature[20].The artery sometimes divides over a short distance in its upper part into two trunks, which join below to form the brachial artery. Often, the artery divides at a higher level than usual, and the vessels involved in this high division are three in number: the radial, the ulnar and the interosseous (IA). Most often, the radial artery divides high up, with the ulnar and interosseous forming the other branch of the bifurcation; in some cases, the ulnar artery arises above the ordinary level, with the radial and interosseous forming the other branch of the division; sometimes, the interosseous artery arises high up. Occasionally, long, thin vessels known as "vasa aberrantia" connect the brachial or axillary arteries to one of the arteries of the forearm, or to branches of these arteries. These vessels generally join the radial artery[20].


## IV. THE ULNAR ARTERY

The ulnar artery, the larger of the two terminal branches of the brachial artery, starts a little below the elbow crease and, passing obliquely downwards, reaches the ulnar side of the forearm at a point roughly midway between the elbow and wrist. It then runs along the ulnar edge to the wrist, crosses the transverse carpal ligament on the radial surface of the pisiform bone and, immediately after this bone, divides into two branches which form the superficial and deep palmar arches.In its upper half, it is deeply buried, covered by the pronator ring muscle, the flexor carpi radialis muscle, the palmaris longus muscle and the deep common flexor muscle of the fingers; it rests on the brachialis muscle and the deep common flexor muscle. The median nerve connects with the medial side of the artery for about 2.5 cm, then crosses the vessel, from which it is separated by the ulnar head of the pronator ring. In the lower half of the forearm, it rests on the deep common flexor, is covered by superficial and deep integument and fascia, and is positioned between the ulnar flexor carpi muscle and the ulnar ring pronator muscle.deep common flexor. It is accompanied by two satellite veins and is overlapped in its middle third by the ulnar flexor carpi; the ulnar nerve lies on the medial side of the lower two-thirds of the artery, and the palmar cutaneous branch of the nerve runs down the lower part of the vessel to the palm of the hand. On the wrist, the ulnar artery is covered by the integument and the palmar carpal ligament, and rests on the transverse carpal ligament. On its medial side lies the pisiform bone and, slightly behind the artery, the ulnar nerve.

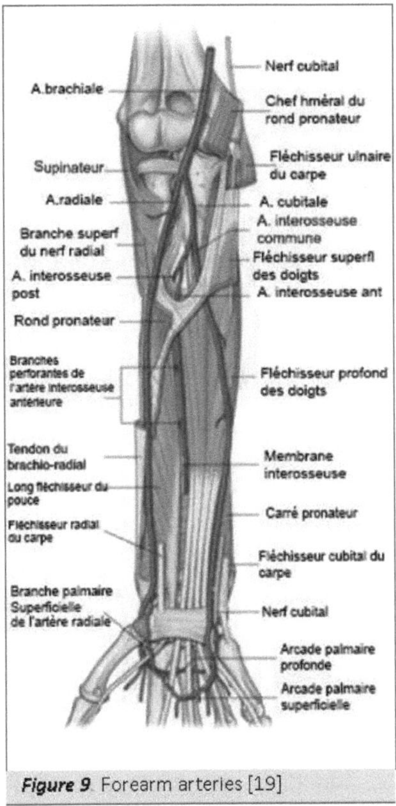



***Figure 9***. Forearm arteries [19]

The origin of the ulnar artery varies in about one in thirteen cases; it may arise some 5 to 7 cm below the elbow, but more frequently higher up. Variations in the position of this vessel are more frequent than those of the radial. When its The vessel's origin is normal, and its course is rarely altered.

When it originates high up, it is almost always superficial to the flexor muscles of the forearm, usually under the fascia, more rarely between the fascia and the integument. In a few cases, its position was subcutaneous in the upper forearm, and subaponeurotic in the lower part[20]. Branches of the ulnar artery arising in the forearm include[19] :

• The recurrent ulnar artery with anterior and posterior branches that contribute to an anastomotic network of vessels around the elbow joint.

• Numerous muscular arteries supply the surrounding muscles;

• The common interosseous artery, which divides into the anterior and posterior interosseous arteries;

• And two small carpal arteries (dorsal carpal branch and palmar carpal branch) supply blood to the wrist.

The posterior interosseous artery runs dorsally along the proximal edge of the interosseous membrane in the posterior compartment of the forearm.

The anterior interosseous artery runs distally along the anterior surface of the interosseous membrane, supplying the muscles of the deep compartment of the forearm, the radius and ulna. It has numerous branches, which perforate the interosseous membrane to supply the deep muscles of the posterior compartment. It also has a small branch that contributes to the vascular network around the carpal bones and joints. Perforating the interosseous membrane in the distal forearm, the anterior interosseous artery terminates by joining the posterior artery.


## V. THE RADIAL ARTERY

The radial artery appears, from its direction, to be a continuation of the brachial artery, but its caliber is smaller than that of the ulnar artery. It starts at the bifurcation of the brachial artery, just below the elbow crease, and runs along the radial surface of the forearm to the wrist. It then wraps back around the lateral surface of the carpus, under the Long abductor and Long and short extensor tendons of the thumb, to the upper end of the space between the metacarpal bones of the thumb and index finger. Finally, it passes forward between the two heads of the first dorsal interosseous, into the palm of the hand, where it crosses the metacarpal bones and, at the ulnar surface of the hand, unites with the deep palmar branch of the ulnar artery to form the deep palmar arch. The radial artery thus has three parts, one in the forearm, one at the back of the wrist and one in the hand. In the forearm, the artery extends from the neck of the radius to the anterior part of the styloid process, lying on the medial side of the body of the bone at the top, and in front of it at the bottom. The upper part of the artery is covered by the ventral fleshy part of the brachioradialis; the rest of the artery is superficial, covered by the integument and superficial aponeuroses. deep. In its downward course, it rests on the Biceps brachii tendon, the supinator, the pronator ring, the radial origin of the deep flexor digitorum communis, the flexor pollicis longus, the pronator quadratus and the lower end of the radius. In the upper third of its course, it lies between the Brachioradialis and the pronator ring; in the lower two-thirds, between the tendons of the Brachioradialis and the flexor carpi radialis. The superficial branch of the radial nerve is close to the lateral side of the artery in the middle third of its course; and a few filaments of the lateral antibrachial cutaneous nerve run along the lower part of the artery as it wraps around the wrist. The vessel is accompanied by a pair of satellite veins all along its course. (See figure 9.)At the wrist, the artery reaches the dorsum carpi, passing between the radial collateral ligament of the wrist and the tendons of the abductor pollicis longus and extensor pollicis brevis. It then descends over the navicular bone and trapezium and, before disappearing between the heads of the first dorsal interosseous, is crossed by the tendon of the long extensor of the thumb.In the hand, it starts at the upper end of the first interosseous space, between the chiefs of the first dorsal interosseous muscle, crosses the palm transversely between the Adductor oblique of the thumb and the Adductor transverse of the thumb, but sometimes pierces the latter muscle, as far as the base of the metacarpal of the little finger, where it anastomoses with the deep palmar branch of the ulnar artery, thus completing the deep palmar arcade[20].In almost one in eight cases, the radial artery originates higher than normal, it more often arises from the axillary or superior part of the brachial artery than from the inferior part of this latter vessel. In the forearm, it deviates from its normal position less often than the ulnar. It has been found resting on the deep fascia rather than under it. It has also been observed on the surface of the brachioradialis muscle, rather than under its medial edge; and on circling the wrist, it has been seen lying on, rather than under, the extensor tendons of the thumb. Branches of the radial artery arising in the forearm include [19]:

• The radial recurrent artery (RRA), which contributes to an anastomotic network around the elbow joint and to numerous vessels supplying the muscles of the lateral aspect of the forearm.
• A small palmar carpal branch, which contributes to an anastomotic network of vessels supplying the bones and joints of the carpus.
• A slightly wider branch, the superficial palmar branch, which enters the hand through, or superficially to, the thenar muscles at the base of the thumb and anastomoses with the superficial palmar arch formed by the ulnar artery.

Given the importance of the radial artery in catheterization procedures, numerous studies have been devoted to it. One interesting study published in 2004 [21] focused on the diameter of this artery, and included 1191 patients from December 1999 to July 2001 with a normal Allen test who underwent transradial coronary angiography, including angioplasty in 275 cases. The mean age of the patients was 60 ±10 years, and 58.4% were men. The internal luminal radial arterial diameter 1 or 2 cm distal to the styloid process, was measured before and after the procedure using two-dimensional ultrasound (10.5 MHz transducer) in 93% of patients (1,103 cases), and retrograde angiography of the radial artery was performed before transradial coronary intervention in all patients. The mean radial arterial diameter was defined as a mean value of the perpendicular internal radial diameter on several occasions. Branch abnormality, radial artery tortuosity and procedural characteristics, including procedure duration and local vascular complications, were also analyzed. The mean arterial diameter on two-dimensional ultrasound was 2.60±0.41 mm, ranging from 1.15 to 3.95 mm (Figure 10). The proportion of mean diameter less than 2.3 mm (outer diameter of 5Fr sheath)was 17.3%; 16.4% were men and 34.4% women. 43.8% had a diameter smaller than the outer diameter of the 6Fr sheath (less than 2.52 mm), of whom 31.7% were men and 59.5% women. 74.4% had a radial artery diameter smaller than the outer diameter of the 7Fr sheath (less than 2.85 mm), of whom 67% were men and 84.9 of women. The average diameter of of the radial artery was significantly correlated with body surface area (r=0.305, p=0.001). There was a significant difference in body surface area (1.72±0.14 vs. 1.53±0.14 m2, p<0.001) and mean diameter (2.69±0.40 vs. 2.43±0.38 mm, p<0.001) between men and women. However, there was no statistical difference between the right and left radial arteries (2.61±0.40 vs. 2.59±0.38 mm)[21].

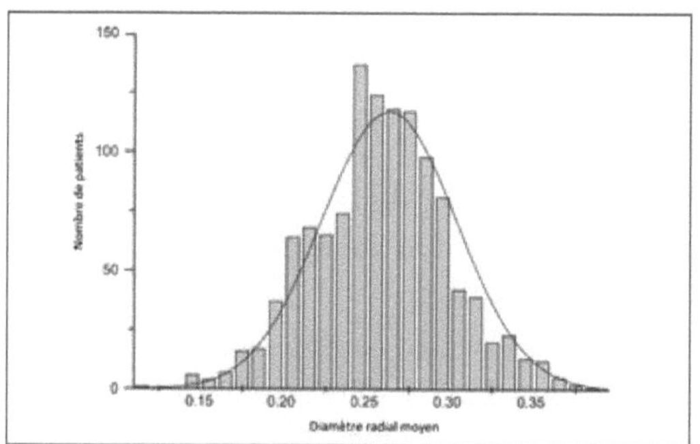


Figure 10. Radial arterial diameter distributions. [21]

Shima et al[22], in a cadaveric study, reported that the mean diameters of the radial artery in the proximal and distal portions were 2.3 and 2.2 mm respectively in a Japanese population, which may explain this slight difference in diameter from the previous series. Nagai et al[23] evaluated the vascular complications of this method by two-dimensional ultrasound and color Doppler studies in 162 patients before, early (2 ±2 days) and late (95 ±29 days) after catheterization. The mean age was 64 ±10 years, and 103 were men. Coronary angioplasty was performed in 59 patients (79 lesions), with angiographic success in 92% of cases. Early in the procedure, segmental stenosis was noted in 35 patients (22%) and no flow in 15 (9%). At the end of the procedure, segmental stenosis was noted in 2 patients, diffuse stenosis in 36 (22%) and no flow in 8 (5%).Thirty-three of 86 patients (38%) with no flow or diffuse stenosis had radial artery diameters less than the introducer diameter, and 11 of 76 patients (14%) had radial artery diameters greater than the sheath diameter (p <0.01). Multivariate analysis revealed risk factors for vascular complications:

• Pre-procedural radial artery diameter was a significant and independent determinant of no flow both early (p = 0.06) and late (p = 0.004) after surgery.
• The difference between radial artery diameter and introducer size was associated with the occurrence of diffuse stenosis at the end of the procedure (p= 0.003).

Thus, ultrasonic assessment of the radial artery was useful in selecting both an appropriate access route and introducer size to avoid early and late vascular complications.


## VI. ANATOMICAL VARIATION OF THE RADIAL ARTERY

Anatomical variations in the radial artery result from the embryological development of the arteries of the upper limb from an initial capillary plexus, proximally to distally.

### 1. Brachioradialis artery

The brachioradial artery (BRA) has been used as a clear, unifying nomenclature for previously used terminology: "high origin of the radial artery", "radial artery from the axillary artery", "high bifurcation of the brachial artery", "continuation of the superficial brachial artery as a radial artery" and "double brachial artery". The brachioradialis artery is a uniform term used to designate the high origin of the radial artery proximal to the elbow from the brachial artery[24] or, less frequently, the axillary artery[25].
R. Haladaj et al[24] have analyzed in detail the anatomical variations of the brachioradial artery in terms of the variability of its origin, the presence and types of anastomosis with the brachial artery in the ulnar fossa ("cubital crossover" or "cubital connection", which is an anastomosing artery that passes

variably between the brachioradial artery and the "normal" brachial artery[24].), and of the pattern of recurrent radial arteries, as well as of the vascular territory within the hand, among the 120 upper limbs examined, the radial artery has a high origin in 11 specimens (11/120; 9.2% of the total number of limbs): six male limbs (6/65; 9.2% of male limbs) and five female limbs (5/55; 9.1% of female limbs). In addition, this variation was found on the right side in six cases (6/63; 9.5% of right limbs) and on the left side in five cases (5/57 ; 8.8% of left limbs). No statistically significant difference was found between the frequency of presence of the brachioradialis artery and sex or side of the body.

An anastomosis between the brachioradialis artery and the conventional brachial arteries in the ulnar fossa, known as the "ulnar crossing" or "ulnar connection", is frequently observed and has several variants:

• Conventional anatomy (figure 11A) without BRA.

• Dominant-type ulnar crossing (Figure 11B) with a hypoplastic pre-anastomotic part of the BRA (~9% of BRAs).

• Balanced-type ulnar crossing (Fig. 11C): anastomosis characterized by a diameter similar to that of the BRA (~27% of BRAs).

• Arterial island (Fig. 11D): in rare cases, two arteries (BRA and brachial artery) may create an arterial complex (like an island) at the level of the radial neck, terminating in a division into radial and ulnar arteries. This extremely rare form has no reported incidence and is limited to isolated case reports.

• Ulnar crossing type

minimal (Fig. 11E): anastomosis with a diameter smaller than that of the ulnar artery (~18% of ulnar arteries).

• Absence of ulnar crossing (Fig. 11F): no anastomosis between the BRA and the conventional brachial artery in the ulnar fossa (~45% of BRAs).

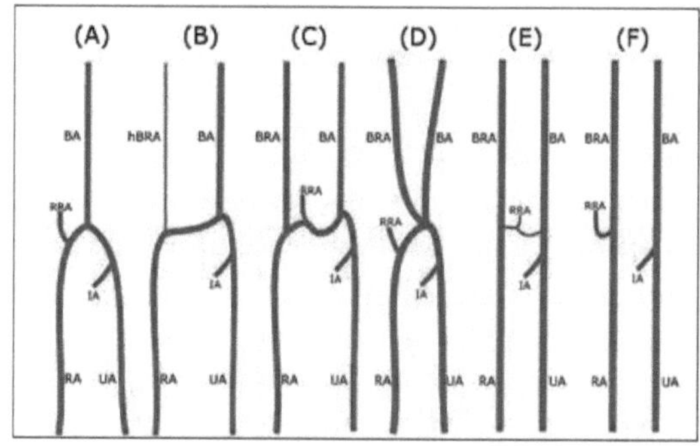


Figure 11. Anatomical variations of the radial artery [25].

BRA is a risk factor for the development of vascular complications during radial access. Given the high prevalence of this atypia (close to 10%), the interventionist using the radial route must discern these variants in order to perform catheterization safely and effectively.

## 2. Loops of the radial artery

Radial artery loops represent a less frequent anatomical variant that can present a significant challenge to the success of the transradial procedure. Dossani et al[26] in a case series, described the anatomy and frequency of radial artery loops and provided a technique for successful navigation of this anatomical anomaly. In this study, a total of 997 transradial approach procedures were performed.

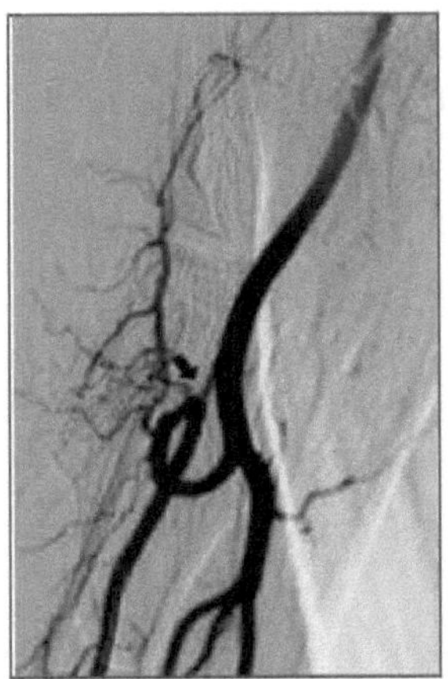

Figure 12. Injection of the right radial artery shows a 3600 loop of the radial artery. [26] performed over a 9-month period. A radial loop was identified in 10 patients (1.0%).

The mean age was 68.6 ±14.3 years. An advanced microcatheter on a 0.014″ guide was used to navigate the loop and avoid entry into the recurrent branch. These loops are located just distal to the origin of the radial artery, and can be characterized either by the classic 360° loop (figure 12), or by a simple, marked tortuosity greater than 90°. The radial artery loop is invariably accompanied by the recurrent radial artery, which follows a straight course in the upper arm (figure 12, black arrow).

### 3. Origin of the radial artery

The radial artery arises 1 cm downstream of the elbow flexion crease as a terminal branch of the brachial artery in the ulnar fossa at the level of the neck of the radius (Figure 9). The radial artery continues in the same direction as its parent trunk and extends from the ulnar fossa to the palm, terminating in an anastomosis with the ulnar artery to form the deep palmar arch, as described above.A low-lying origin of the radial artery is a rare anatomical variation, with an estimated incidence of 0.2%. Wysiadecki et al[27] reported a novel case of an unusual distal origin of the radial artery, coinciding with a recurrent double radial artery. The radial artery originated beneath the rond pronator muscle, 76 mm below the intercondylar line of the humerus. After emerging beneath the tendon of the round pronator muscle, it followed a typical course and terminated in the deep palmar arch.

### 4. Absence of the radial artery

Absence of the radial artery has been reported rarely, with an estimated incidence of less than 0.2%. In these cases, the radial blood supply was provided by the anterior interosseous artery or the medial artery[28].

### 5. The superficial radial artery

The superficial radial artery is a radial artery that passes over the tendons defining the snuffbox. It is a rare finding, affecting around 0.4% of adult upper limbs. It may adopt its superficial course at different levels of the forearm; the distal superficial course being considered the most frequent[28].


## VII. ANATOMY OF THE DISTAL RADIAL AND THE HAND

In the wrist and hand, the radial and ulnar arteries create a dense anastomotic network that ensures arterial blood flow to the hand (Figure 13). These arteries are located on the palmar surface of the hand and comprise the deep palmar arcade and the superficial palmar arcade[29]. The ulnar artery continues across the palm in the form of the superficial palmar arcade, which is variably supplemented by a branch from the radial artery. Distally, the radial artery gives rise to the palmar carpal branch to form a transverse anastomosis with the homologous branch from the ulnar artery and the superficial palmar branch, which passes through the thenar muscles, sometimes anastomosing with the tip of the ulnar artery to complete the superficial palmar arcade.

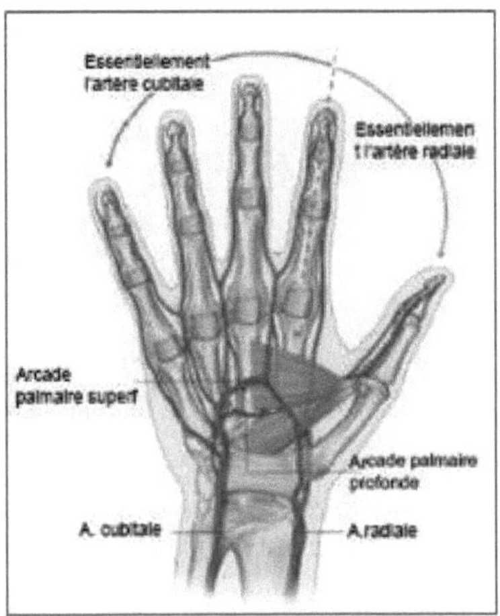



**Figure 13.** Arterial irrigation of the hand. [19]

At the wrist, the radial artery curves posterolaterally.to pass over the dorsal surface of the carpus between the long extensor tendon of the thumb and the long abductor tendons and the extensor digitorum brevis,      crossing obliquely over the scaphoid bone and trapezium into the anatomical snuffbox, where its pulse is usually evident (figure14). Above the trapezium, the radial artery gives rise to the dorsal branch of the carpus forms, with its ulnar counterpart, the dorsal arch of the carpal arteries supplying the dorsal metacarpal arteries and the radiodorsal digital artery of the thumb. A pulse can also be felt on the back of the hand, at the apex of the angle between the long extensor tendon of the thumb and the second metacarpal, as the radial artery travels medially between the heads of the first dorsal interosseous muscle in the palm, where it anastomoses with the deep branch of the ulnar artery, completing the deep palmar arcade. Blood supply to the fingers is mainly provided by the interconnected palmar metacarpal arteries and the common palmar digital arteries, which arise from the deep and superficial palmar arches respectively.

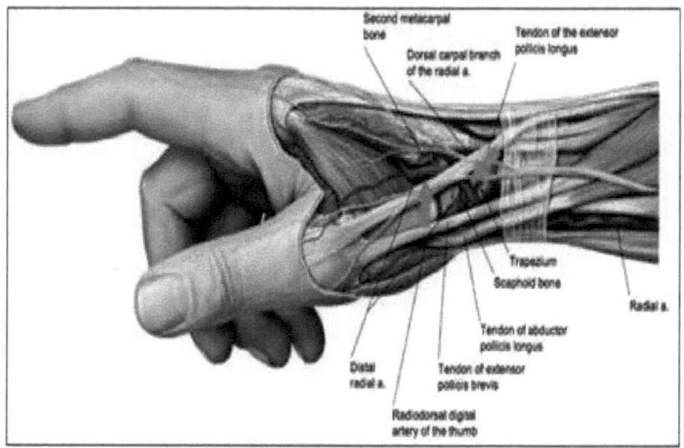



Figure 14. Distal radial artery puncture sites (blue arrows) and surrounding anatomical structures [30].

Although the blood supply to the hand has been studied by many investigators, the substantial variability in the anatomy of the superficial and deep palmar arches seems to be the only consistent finding. Jaschtschinski[30] in 1897 initially subdivided the superficial palmar arch into 2 types: complete and incomplete (figure 15). This classification is still useful today for identifying patients whose anastomotic network is potentially insufficient to tolerate radial artery ligation.

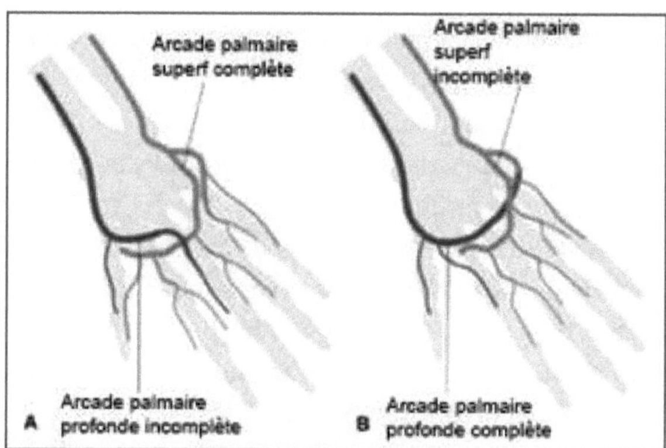



Figure15. Vascularization complete and incomplete vascularization of the hand [30].

Theoretically, a patient with a complete superficial and deep palmar arch should be able to tolerate ligation of the radial or ulnar artery, as collateral flow will preserve perfusion of the radial or ulnar artery, thus improving the quality of blood flow. Conversely, occlusion of the radial artery in a patient with 2 incomplete arches could significantly increase the risk of The superficial palmar arcade is defined as complete when it vascularizes all the fingers including the ulnar side of the thumb, and the deep palmar arcade is defined as complete when the tip of the radial artery is connected to the deep palmar branch of the ulnar artery. Recent agiographic studies have shown that the superficial palmar arcade was incomplete in 46% of cases, whereas the deep palmar arcade was complete in all patients[31].

# DISTAL TRANSRADIAL ACCESS: THE SCIENCE BEHIND THE TECHNIQUE

## I. FEASIBILITY

There's no denying that, as a new technique, DRA faces a number of challenges. The first and most important is the success rate of the puncture. The diameter of the artery in the anatomical snuffbox is smaller than that in the forearm. In addition, the artery is more tortuous, which can reduce the success rate of the puncture. For this reason, many operators believe that there is a certain learning curve, and have suggested that this procedure should be performed by well-trained operators[32]. One of the first studies on the feasibility of DRA was published in 2018 and conducted from October 2017 to February 2018, patients with palpable left distal radial arteries scheduled for coronary angiography or angioplasty were prospectively recruited. Endpoints were success and complication rates. Fifty-six patients were recruited over a 4-week period. Mean age was $64.3 \pm 13.3$ (median: 62) years, with more men (n=38, 67.9%) than women (n=18, 32.1%). Acute coronary syndrome (myocardial infarction: n=18, 32.2%; unstable angina: n=19, 33.9%) was the most frequent condition, followed by stable angina (n=7, 12.5%). Ad hoc angioplasty was performed in 29 patients (52%), and diagnostic coronary angiography in 27 (48%). Two cases of failed puncture (3.57%) by left DRA were observed. When puncture was successful, coronary angiography and ad hoc angioplasty were successful. In this study there were no serious bleeding complications or nerve damage, and it demonstrated good feasibility and safety of DRA[33].

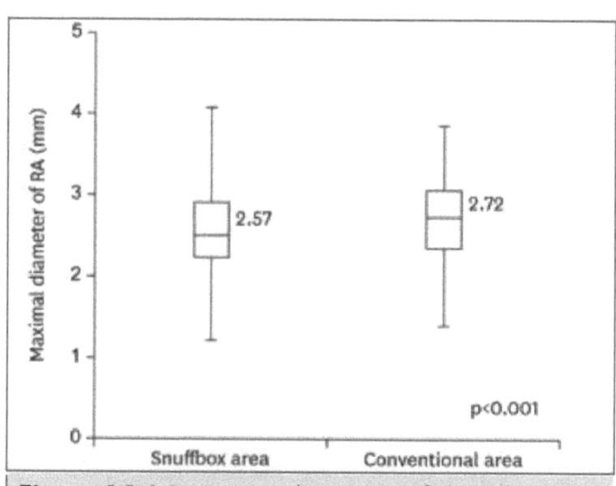


**Figure 16.** Maximum diameter of the tabatière artery and the conventional radial artery [35].

In another study published in 2018 the left distal radial artery was used as an access site in 54 patients admitted for coronary angiography and angioplasty between May 25 and October 20, 2017. All these patients had a distal left radial pulse. The mean age of the patients was 59.3 years, and 80% of them were men. Seventeen patients were admitted for acute coronary syndrome. All underwent successful coronary angiography and left distal transradial angioplasty with Judkins 6 French catheters. Primary angioplasty was performed in 10 patients. A total of 20 patients underwent angioplasty, 11 of them on the interventricular artery. spasm. Two patients experienced brachial spasm requiring right femoral passage. There were no cases of radial artery occlusion, hematoma or hand numbness. Hemostasis was achieved by manual compression. This study concludes that the left distal radial approach is safe and feasible as a new technique for coronary angiography and angioplasty[34]. Also in 2018 Kim et al[35] tried the distal radial approach via the left snuffbox in 150 patients admitted for angiography and/or angioplasty for suspected myocardial ischemia between November 1, 2017 and March 31, 2018. The success rate of distal radial artery cannulation was 88.0% (n=132). Of the 132 individuals, 58 (43.9%) patients had acute coronary syndrome (ACS). The diameter of the artery at the snuffbox was significantly smaller than that of the conventional artery (2.57 mm vs. 2.72 mm, p<0.001) (figure16). However, coronary angiography using a 6-French catheter was successfully performed in all 132 patients. In addition, there was a significant correlation between artery diameter at the snuffbox and that of the conventional (r=0.856, p<0.001). With regard to vascular complications, swelling of the forearm with bruising, which did not require surgery or transfusion, occurred in 2 (4.9%) cases. This study also concludes that the distal radial approach at the level of the left snuffbox is more suitable for coronary angiography and angioplasty than the conventional radial approach. Aoi et al[36] recruited 202 consecutive patients who underwent coronary angiography and angioplasty with distal radial access compared with 206 cases with conventional access. Of the 408 patients, radial access was successfully achieved in 99.5% (201/202) of DRA cases and in 99.0% (204/206) of conventional access cases. The right distal radial artery was accessed in 176 cases (87.6%). Mean access time from local anesthesia to radial flushing was 7.3 minutes. Ninety cases (44.8%) were percutaneous coronary interventions, and the mean dose of heparin used was 4,448 units. The mean time to remove the compression band was 104.7 min (120.8 min for angioplasty and 91.7 min for diagnosis). The follow-up ultrasound study showed two partial occlusions (1.0%) and one arteriovenous fistula (0.5%). They concluded that despite the longer time to access the distal radial artery in the anatomical snuffbox, this is a safe and feasible alternative to the conventional radial route, which could reduce hemostasis time, particularly in cases of angioplasty.The DISCORADIAL trial [37] involving over 1309 patients compared the impact of the distal approach on the procedure, in terms of major complications such as radial artery occlusion and haematomas, as well as puncture time, ease of inserting the stent, patient comfort, procedure duration and time to haemostasis. The study found an exceptionally low rate of radial artery occlusion, with a rate three times lower in the distal radial group, a significantly shorter hemostasis time and a lower incidence of bleeding complications. However, these advantages are counterbalanced by a longer approach time. slightly longer and a higher rate of switch to RCA due to the small caliber of the artery[37].As shown by other studies with sample sizes greater than 20, the success rate varies between 70% and 100%[32]. In the two largest studies, the success rate was 99.7% for 1631 patients and 97% for 2696 patients[38], [39].Recently li et al[40] in a study published in 2023 explored the feasibility and safety of distal transradial access in patients with acute chest pain, i.e. in an emergency setting. A total of 1269 patients complaining of acute chest pain were retrospectively included from January 2020 to February 2022. Patients who met the inclusion criteria were divided into the conventional transradial access group (n = 238) and the DRA group (n = 158). Propensity score matching was used to minimize baseline differences. The cannulation success rate in the ARD group was significantly lower than in the ARC group (87.41% vs. 94.81%, p < 0,05). There was no significant difference between the two groups in puncture time or total procedure time (p > 0.05). Compared with the ARC group, the duration of hemostasis was significantly shorter [4(4, 4) h vs. 10(8, 10) h, p < 0.001) and the incidence of minor bleeding (BARC Type I and II) was significantly lower in the ARD group than in the ARC group (0.85% vs. 5.48%, p = 0.045). Asymptomatic radial artery occlusion was observed in six patients (5.83%) in the ARC group and in one patient (1.14%) in the ARD group (p = 0.126). Analysis of the ST-segment elevation myocardial infarction (STEMI) subgroup showed no significant differences in puncture time, Door-to-Balloon time or total procedure time between the two groups. In conclusion, DRA for coronary angiography or emergency angioplasty has an acceptable success rate and puncture time, a shorter hemostasis time and a trend towards a lower radial occlusion rate than ARC. DRA did not increase the Door-to- Balloon ratio.

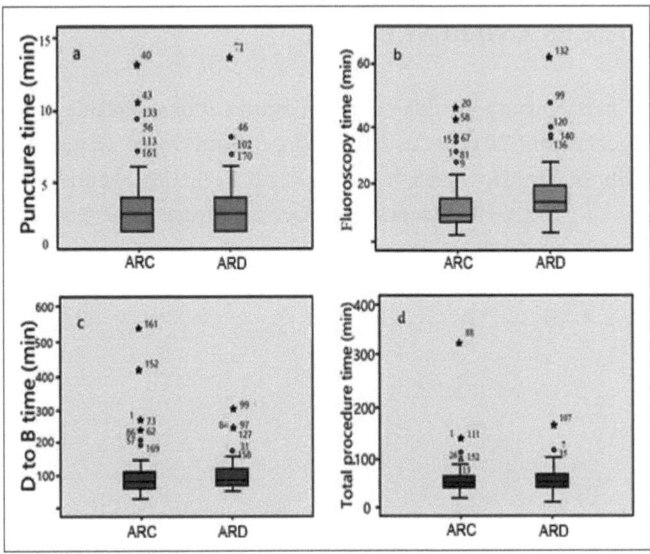

Figure 17. Comparison of delays associated with emergency procedures in patients with ST-segment elevation myocardial infarction [40].

Interestingly, only one randomized study reported that the success rate of the distal radial was less than 80%, which was significantly lower than that of the conventional radial[41]. However, we must be aware that certain factors can affect results. The first is the success criterion. In some studies, success was defined when the needle was inserted into the vessel, while in others, success was catheter insertion. For example, Kim. Y. reported that the success rate was 93.3% according to the former definition, but only 88.0% according to the latter definition [35].Puncture methods also affect the success rate. Some operators have used the "anterior wall puncture" technique [15], while others prefer a transfixing puncture of the artery [35]. Given that the carpal bones lie just below the artery, and that puncturing the periosteum causes significant pain, transfixing puncture is not recommended by some interventionists.

## II. ADVANTAGES AND BENEFITS

1. Impact on radial artery occlusion and complications vascular Occlusion of radial artery occlusion (RAO) is usually asymptomatic and does not affect quality of life of quality of life. However, it is of interest to the interventionist, as it may be necessary to repeat the access for another procedure. The distal radial approach not only prevents occlusion of the radial artery; it is also the principal site of recanalization retrograde occlusion of the latter.

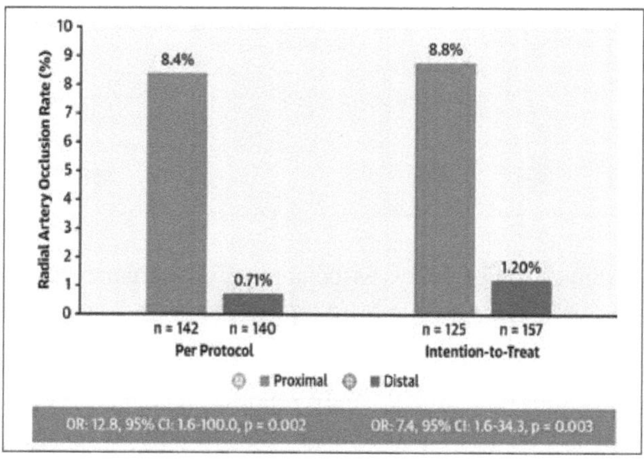


Figure 18. Rate of proximal radial artery occlusion at 24 hours by ARC or ARD [42].

Eid-Lidt et al[42] conducted a prospective, comparative, longitudinal, randomized study to compare the rate of proximal radial artery occlusion using Doppler ultrasound between distal radial access and conventional radial access 24 hours and 30 days after a transradial coronary procedure. A total of 282 patients were randomized between proximal radial access (n = 142) and distal radial access (n = 140) to assess the superiority of the distal approach in preventing proximal radial artery occlusion. In the per-protocol analysis, proximal radial artery occlusion rates at 24 h and 30 days were 8.4% and 5.6% respectively in the proximal group, and 0.7% and 0.7% in the distal group (24 h: odds ratio [OR]: 12.8; 95% confidence interval [CI]: 1.6 to 100.0; p = 0.002; 30 days: OR: 8.2; 95% CI: 1.0 to 67.2; p = 0.019). In an intention-to-treat analysis, occlusion rates at 24 hours and 30 days were 8.8% and 6.4% for proximal radial access and 1.2% and 0.6% in the distal radial access group (24 h: OR: 7.4; 95%

CI: 1.6 to 34.3; p = 0.003; 30 days: OR: 10.6; 95% CI: 1.3 to 86.4; p = 0.007). This study clearly shows that distal radial access prevents occlusion in the proximal segment 24 hours and 30 days after surgery, compared with conventional radial access (figure 18).The study by Alexander Achim et al [43] published in December 2021 was a large multicenter study aimed at facilitating the widespread use of the distal radial by proving not only its feasibility and low complication rate, but also its impact on the duration of the approach as well as the duration of the complete procedure. This study showed a small group of patients were exposed to benign complications such as hematoma in 0.32% of cases, arterial dissection in 0.4% of cases and distal occlusion in 0.4% of patients. It should be noted that follow-up of patients with radial occlusions showed repermeabilization one month after the event, explained by better development of collaterals distal to the artery. These data point to a very low complication rate. Furthermore, the study showed that, after a relatively short learning curve (15 cases on average), the impact of the change of strategy on the duration of the approach and on the overall duration of the procedure was low, with no additional exposure to radiation or use of contrast medium[43]. Mizuguchi et al[44] in their study attempted to investigate the effects of DRA use on radial artery occlusion and post-procedural bleeding. From April 2018 to July 2018, 228 consecutive patients undergoing coronary angiography or intervention via DRA at two hospitals were analyzed. Radial occlusion rate, forearm and distal radial artery diameter change and cross-sectional area after DRA (at 1 day and 1 month) on vascular ultrasound, and incidence of bleeding complications were studied. Radial forearm occlusion and distal occlusion occurred in 1 (0.4%) and 8 (3.1%) patients at 1 month, respectively. No forearm hematomas occurred. Ultrasonographic findings indicated that radial artery diameter and cross-sectional area were significantly larger after DRA (2.9 ± 0.5 mm vs. 2.7± 0.5 mm, p < 0.001 and 6.5 ± 2.4 $mm^2$ vs. 5.6 ± 2.0 $mm^2$, p < 0.001, respectively). Distal radial artery diameter and cross-sectional area in the anatomical snuffbox were also significantly greater after DRA (2.5 ± 0.5 mm vs. 2.3 ± 0.4 mm, p < 0.001 and 4.7 ± 2.0 $mm^2$ vs. 4.2 ± 1.6 $mm^2$, p < 0.001, respectively). DRA was associated with a low incidence of radial occlusion at the puncture site and in the forearm, post-procedural dilatation of the radial artery and absence of hemorrhagic complications extending to the forearm.

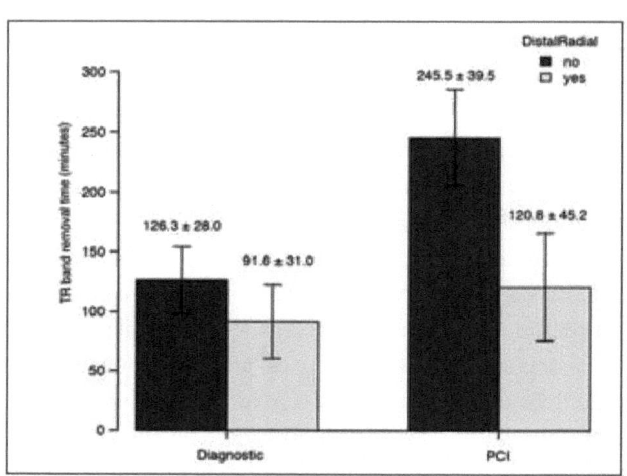


Figure 19. Comparison of compression band removal time between DRA and CRA stratified by procedure type (diagnostic catheterization vs angioplasty)[36].

2. Impact on duration of compression and hemostasis

In the study by Aoi et al[36] hemostasis time was significantly shorter for DRA in the anatomical snuffbox than for CRA: around 30 minutes less for diagnostic catheterization and 60 minutes less for angioplasty. Angioplasty cases inevitably had a longer hemostasis time due to the higher dose of heparin; however, this study interestingly showed that angioplasty cases with distal radial access had a hemostasis time similar to that of diagnostic catheterization with conventional radial access (figure 19). Previous studies have shown that early control of hemostasis was achieved in less than 3 hours. The smaller size of the vessel distal to the bifurcation, the superficial position and the anatomical position on a bony base are plausible explanations for this finding. Faster haemostasis without increased risk of complication is clinically significant in terms of post-procedural care and patient comfort, and also economically significant since same-day discharge has been shown to deliver substantial cost savings. Sanhoury et al[45] randomized one hundred cases with varying indications for coronary intervention into two groups using systematic random sampling. Coronary interventions in the first group were performed by ARD (50 patients) and in the second group by ARC (50 patients). Post-procedural compression time in group I was 2.0-7.0 with a mean standard deviation of 5.14 ± 0.88, while post-procedural compression time in group II was 19.0-40.0 with a mean standard deviation of 24.50 ± 4.02 P= 0.001 indicates that there were statistically significant differences between the groups. We should point out that post-procedural manual compression was used in Group I patients, while radial taping was used in Group II patients, denoting the major advantage of the ARD approach in post-procedural hemostasis. So, we conclude that since the artery is small and superficial, with a bony platform underneath; hemostasis does not require too much pressure from the compression device or bandage. In addition, compression time is significantly shorter with the ARD than with the ATR.

3. Patient and physician comfort

The distal radial technique seems to offer more advantages. Firstly, the position of the arm during the procedure is comfortable for the patient, who does not have to expose the palmar aspect of the arm while flexing the upper arm towards the operator, as the left hand is placed close to the groin, with the back facing upwards. No equipment or investment is required to support the patient's left arm. Another advantage for the patient is that, if he or she is right-handed, the use of the dominant upper limb is no longer restricted during the hemostatic compression that follows catheter removal[15]. This same left-arm position may also be appreciated by operators who have been trained in transfemoral access and prefer the left approach to coronary arteries. The operator can work as usual on the patient's right side and does not need to bend over the patient to reach the left radial artery.

## III. DISTAL TRANSRADIAL ACCESS IN CHRONIC OCCLUSIONS

This approach has proved particularly suitable for procedures requiring a double vascular approach, such as CTO. In a study by Nikolakopoulos et al, comparing the distal and proximal approaches in a series of 120 CTOs performed as part of the PROGRESS-CTO registry[46], the success rate was found to be similar in both groups (90% ARD vs. 86% ARC; P=.14), as was the complication rate (0.8% ARD vs. 2.4% ARC; P=.26), with a lower rate of tamponade requiring pericardiosynthesis (0% ARD vs 4.69% ARC; P<.001), as did the air kerma radiation dose (median, 1.7 Gy; interquartile range [IQR], 0.97- 2.63 Gy in the ARD group vs median, 2.27 Gy; IQR, 1.2-3.9 Gy in the ARC group; P<0.001). [46]. So for the distal radial approach in a CTO context, in addition to the success rate which is practically the same as other approaches, there are advantages for the patient in terms of comfort and advantages for the physician in terms of comfort too and above all in terms of reduced exposure to ryonement, these results were confirmed in another recent study ( published in 2022) where Achim et al.[47] compared safety and feasibility in angioplasty of chronic total occlusions (CTO) by DRA, From 2016 to 2021, all patients undergoing CTO in 3 Hungarian centers were included, divided into 2 groups: one benefiting from conventional radial access and the other from DRA. Primary endpoints were procedural and clinical success and complications related to vascular access. Secondary endpoints were major adverse cardiac and cerebrovascular events (MACCE) and procedural characteristics (contrast volume, fluoroscopy time, radiation dose, procedure duration, hospital stay). A total of 337 consecutive patients (mean age $64.6 \pm 9.92$ years, 72.4% male) were enrolled (ARC = 257, ARD = 80). Compared with ARD, the ARC group had a higher prevalence of smoking (53.8% vs. 25.7%, SMD = 0.643), family history of cardiovascular disease (35.0% vs. 15.2%, SMD = 0.553) and dyslipidemia (95.0% vs. 72.8%, SMD = 0.500). CTO complexity was slightly higher in the ARD group, with higher degrees of calcification and tortuosity, more bifurcation lesions (45.0% vs. 13.2%, MDS = 0.938), more proximal cap ambiguity (67.5% vs. 47.1 %, SMD = 0.409). Contrast volumes (median 120 ml vs. 146 ml, p = 0.045) and dose area (median 928 mGy×cm² vs. 1,300 mGy×cm², p < 0.001) were lower in the ARD group. Numerically, local vascular complications were more frequent in the ARD group, although not statistically significant (RAO 2.72% vs. 1.25%, p = 0.450; large hematoma: 0.72% vs. 0%, p = 1.000). Hospital stay was similar (2.5 vs. 3.0 days, p = 0.4). Procedural and clinical success rates were comparable between ARD and ARC (p = 0.6), and the 12-month MACCE rate was similar in the 2 groups (9.09% vs. 18.2%, p = 0.35). In terms of radiation protection, the lower surface dose product with ARD in this study (a 34% reduction vs. ARC in matched analyses) is encouraging. In this respect, DRA may help to effectively address one of the main disadvantages of traditional radial access compared to transfemoral access, namely greater exposure to radiation. Ultimately, placing both hands above the patient's pelvis is equivalent to transfemoral positioning.

# IV. DISTAL TRANSRADIAL ACCESS IN NON-CORONARY INDICATIONS

## 4. TAVI

As in the case of CTO, the use of the distal radial as a second vascular approach for percutaneous coronary angiography (PCI) is also an option. Transcatheter Aortic Valve Implantation (TAVI) has been proven without complications in a recent study published in July 2022, in which a radial   radial distal approach as a secondary access site for TAVI was adopted. The primary endpoints were technical success and major adverse events (MACCE). Secondary endpoints: access site complication rate, hemodynamic and clinical outcomes of the procedure, procedure-related factors, rate of switch to femoral access and hospital stay (in days). Since November 2020, 41 patients have undergone TAVI using this strategy. Patients had a mean age of $76 \pm 11.2$ years, 41% were male. Six (14.63%) patients received a balloon-expandable valve and 35 (85.37%) a self-expandable valve. The procedure was successful in all cases. No complications arose from transradial access. Puncture success, defined as complete catheter placement, was maximum (N = 41/41, 100%), and secondary transfemoral access was not required in any case. Complications at the site of primary transfemoral vascular access occurred in 7 cases (17%), of which 4 (13.63%) were resolved by distal radial access: one occlusion, two flow-limiting stenoses and four perforations of the common femoral artery. There were no other major vascular complications at 30 days. The overall MACCE rate was 2.4%. The authors concluded that the use of the distal radial approach for secondary access in TAVI is safe, feasible and has several advantages over previous access sites[48].

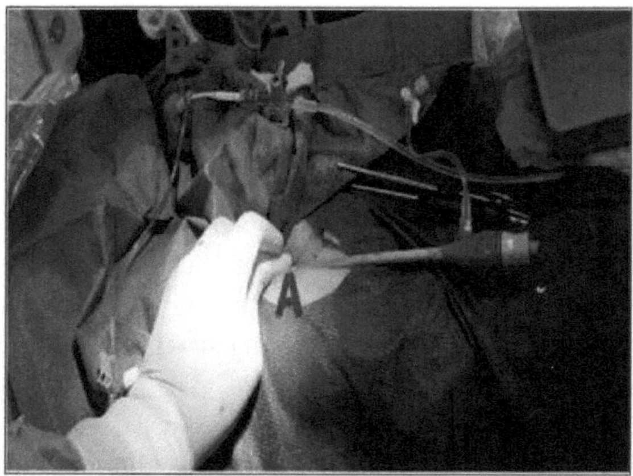

Figure 20. patient example, right femoral primary access (A) and left distal radial secondary access (B), with both sheaths in close proximity to each other, improving ergonomics and reducing radiation dose. [47]

5. Neurovascular interventions

Neuroendovascular procedures have traditionally been performed via the transfemoral route. Transradial access has recently gained popularity due to its lower rate of access-site complications, faster recovery time and greater patient satisfaction. However, ATR is not free of complications, including radial artery occlusion, hematoma, vasospasm. Distal transradial access with radial artery puncture in the anatomical snuffbox may be safer than proximal transradial access, although there are numerous reports on the safety and efficacy of ATR for coronary angiography and percutaneous coronary interventions, data regarding this approach for neuroendovascular procedures are scarce and have not been reviewed. In 2018, McCarthy et al[49] reported for the first time successful experiences in two patients. One underwent only cervical angiography using a 5 Fr catheter, and the other underwent mechanical thrombectomy and balloon angioplasty of the basilar artery using a 0.088″ INFINITY guide catheter. No access-related complications were observed. Al Saiegh et al[50] successfully implanted the Woven EndoBridge device in a woman with an anterior communicating aneurysm via the ARD. Two retrospective studies involving 116 patients undergoing diagnostic cerebral angiography were published in 2019[51],[52] The total success rate of cannulation via the DRA in these studies was 90.52%. A non-randomized study including 58 cases via ARD and 151 via ATR was conducted to explore the feasibility and safety of the new carotid intervention technique using a 6.5Fr JR5 sheathless guiding[53]. The success rate of the procedure was not significantly different in the ARD group (100%) and the ATR group (94%). In contrast to the ATR group, fluoroscopy and procedure times were significantly higher in the ARD group. However, there was no difference in contrast medium consumption and cumulative X-ray dose between the two groups. Only one case of AV fistula requiring surgical reconstruction in the ARD group and two cases of asymptomatic radial artery occlusion in the ATR group.A very recent study, published in March 2023 by Di Gioia, et al.[54] who investigated whether a systematic distal radial approach using 5 Fr guiding catheters was a safe and effective alternative to the trans-femoral approach for stenting the carotid artery. From July 2020 to October 2022, two operators in this study systematically performed carotid angioplasty using a 5 Fr distal radial approach in consecutive patients. The study's primary endpoints were procedural success using the distal radial approach and the proximal or distal radial approach. The learning curve was assessed by comparing the first half of patients with the second half of enrolled patients. Procedural data and clinical results at 30 days were collected. Fifty-one patients were prospectively enrolled. Carotid angioplasty was performed effectively via distal radial access in 45 patients (88%). The overall success rate for the radial artery was 92%. Distal radial angioplasty was successfully performed in 20 of the first 25 patients enrolled (80%) and in 25 of the last 26 patients enrolled (96%; p = 0.07). Significantly less contrast was administered in the last 26 patients versus the first 25 (110 (70, 140) ml versus 120 (107, 150) ml; p = 0.045). Radial artery occlusion was reported in one patient (2%). Only one minor stroke (2%) was reported in hospital and at 30-day follow-up. This study shows that carotid angioplasty via the distal radial using 5 Fr catheters was a safe procedure with a high success rate. It also highlights the importance of the procedure's learning curve, which was relatively short for operators accustomed to the trans-femoral route. Hoffman et al[55] in a study aimed at carrying out a systematic review and meta-analysis of DRA for cerebral angiography and percutaneous neurological interventions, pooled a total of 7 studies comprising 348 (75.8%) diagnostic cerebral angiograms and 111 (24.2%) interventions meeting the inclusion criteria. The pooled success rate was 95% (95% CI, 91%-98%; $I2$ = 74.33). The pooled rate of minor complications was 2% (95% CI, 1%-4%; $I2$ = 0). No major complications were reported. For diagnostic procedures, the combined mean fluoroscopy time was 13.53 [SD, 8.82] minutes and the mean contrast dose was 74.9 [SD, 35.6] ml. The authors concluded that this early experience with distal transradial access suggests that it is a safe and effective alternative to proximal radial and femoral access for performing angiography and diagnostic brain procedures.

The limitations of this systematic review are:

• A small number of studies met the inclusion criteria,
• All were retrospective
• None compared results w i t h  conventional transradial or proximal femoral access.

Further studies are needed to establish its effectiveness and compare it with other access sites.


6. Perioperative


Arterial cannulation is an invasive procedure commonly performed in operating theatres, intensive care units and emergency departments. Arterial cannulation enables real-time blood pressure measurement, blood sampling for blood gas analysis, and can be used to guide therapy (vascular filling) in critically ill patients or those who have undergone surgery. Maitra et al[56] tested the safety and feasibility of distal radial artery cannulation at the anatomical snuffbox perioperatively in adult patients undergoing elective surgery. In this retrospective cohort study, data from 55 patients were examined; of these, 21 patients underwent ultrasound-guided arterial puncture and 34 patients underwent palpation-guided puncture of the distal radial artery at the anatomical snuffbox. The success rate for the first attempt at distal radial arterial cannulation was 76.3% (42 of 55 patients), and was similar between the ultrasound-guided and palpation-guided techniques (P = 0.53). Overall, the success rate of The rate of cannulation was 87.3% (48 of 55 patients), and was also similar between the ultrasound-guided technique and the palpation technique (P = 0.79). This shows that this technique is feasible for patients undergoing elective surgery.

7. Other


Interventionalists may consider distal radial puncture not only as an access site for coronary angiography, but also as an option for the endovascular management of acute upper limb ischemia in cases of embolism of cardiac origin. Giusca, et al[57] published the desperate case of an 83-year-old woman who presented with acute upper limb ischemia due to thrombotic occlusion of the left brachial artery. At the same time, the patient was diagnosed with atrial fibrillation and was not being treated with oral anticoagulation. Trans-femoral thrombectomy using a Rotarex® 6F catheter removed the thrombus from the brachial artery. However, significant amounts of debris embolized distally, causing occlusion of the radial and ulnar arteries. The debris was successfully removed after puncture of the distal radial artery and retrograde aspiration of the thrombus using an Envoy 5F catheter. This maneuver restored flow in the radial and ulnar arteries and completely resolved the patient's ischemic symptoms.A 2017 study[58] shows that this approach can also be used for visceral procedures, with 50 visceral interventional procedures performed in 31 patients, including liver embolotherapy, visceral arterial stent insertion, aneurysm embolization and emergency embolization. In all cases, the procedures were successfully completed using snuffbox access, with only one case of asymptomatic pseudoaneurysm as the only access-related complication. Initial experience has shown that radial access at snuffbox level is technically feasible and represents a viable alternative to conventional radial access for visceral interventional procedures.

# TECHNICAL

Distal transradial access is a relatively simple and safe technique, but requires careful preoperative preparation and assessment.

## I. PREOPERATIVE EVALUATION

### 1. Test d'Allen

The most frequent complication associated with transradial access is radial artery occlusion, which occurs in 1% to 12% of cases. Although considered a rare event, acute hypoperfusion of certain parts of the hand has devastating consequences, such as partial necrosis of the fingers.The Allen test is used to assess collateral blood flow in the hands, in particular to check for the presence of a complete palmar arch[59], usually in preparation for a procedure likely to disrupt blood flow in the radial or ulnar arteries. It was first described in 1929 by Edgar Van Nuys Allen[60]. A negative Allen test means that the patient probably does not have an adequate double blood supply to the hand, which may constitute a contraindication to the planned procedure or at least suggest that further evaluation is required. In 1952, Irving Wright described a modified version of the Allen test which has since largely supplanted the original method[61].Originally, it is performed by asking the patient to raise both arms above the head for thirty seconds to exsanguinate the hands. The patient then clenches his hands into a tight fist, and the examiner occludes the radial artery simultaneously on both hands. The patient then quickly opens both hands and the examiner compares the color of the palms. The initial pallor should be replaced by normal hand color as the ulnar arteries re-establish perfusion. The test is then repeated, occluding the ulnar rather than the radial arteries. The time it takes for normal color to return indicates the degree of collateral blood flow. The test is positive when there is a return to normal color in both hands upon occlusion of either artery. Persistent paleness in the palm indicates inadequate collateral blood flow.The modified Allen test differs from the original Allen test mainly in that it examines the radial and/or ulnar arteries on one hand, then repeats the examination on the other side, if necessary. Traditionally, this is performed by first asking the patient to flex the arm at the elbow and then clench the fist to exsanguinate the hand. The ulnar and radial arteries are then simultaneously compressed by the examiner's thumbs. The elbow is extended to a maximum of 180 degrees, avoiding over-extension which could lead to a false-negative test. The fist is then unclenched and the palm should appear white. Compression is then released at the level of the ulnar artery, while maintaining pressure on the radial artery. Once the compression is released, the color should return to the palm, usually within 10 seconds. The test is repeated on the same hand, first releasing the radial artery and continuing to compress the ulnar artery if assessment of radial collateral blood flow is required. In a patient with normal, patent arteries, the color of the palms should return relatively quickly (within 10 seconds, unless the patient is cold) after the release of either artery. If pallor persists in the palm after the fist is unclenched and one of the arteries has been released, the test is negative and indicates an occlusion in the artery that is released.

2. Test Barbeau

The Barbeau test (BT) is another method described by Gérald R. Barbeau (2004) for assessing hand collateral circulation[62]. BT depends on the use of pulse oximetry plethysmography waveforms, which are generally available on every bedside cardiac monitor. Plethysmography waveforms cannot be displayed without sufficient blood supply to the extremities being assessed. The technique involves placing a pulse oximeter on the thumb prior to compression to obtain a baseline saturation and waveform. The examiner then compresses the radial and ulnar arteries until the waveform disappears and the oxygen saturation drops to zero. The pressure on the ulnar artery is then released. Waveform and saturation are recorded before and immediately after compression of the radial artery for up to 2 minutes. The 2-minute period was chosen arbitrarily. If these values conform to the baseline, collateral flow is good[63]. Plethysmographic readings were divided into 4 types:

• A, no damping of the pulse trace immediately after compression of the radial artery;
• B, pulse trace damping ;
• C, loss of pulse trace followed by restoration of pulse trace within 2 minutes ;
• D, loss of pulse tracing without recovery within 2 minutes.

Oximetry (SpO2) results were either positive (reading present and constant) or negative during radial artery compression (Figure 21).

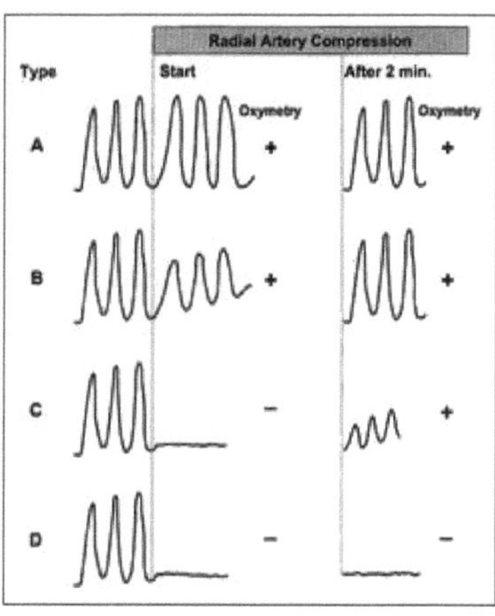


Figure 21. The 4 types of ulnopalmar arch patency results [62].

The presence of a pulse during compression of the radial artery, as in types A and B, represents uninterrupted pulsatile arterial filling. Since a radial artery pulse may be present in the case of radial artery occlusion with a permeable palmar arch in many cases, the differentiation between types A and B unmasks the radial artery occlusion that is sometimes observed in type A; in this case, compression of the radial artery does not reduce pulsatile blood flow at the level of the radial artery. of the thumb. Occlusion of the radial artery can then be suspected when compression of the ulnar artery produces a type D result, allowing assessment of radial artery patency before and after the procedure. In the case of type C, pulsatile blood flow and pulse oximetry are temporarily abolished by radial artery compression, but reappear within a predetermined period of time, arbitrarily chosen as 2 minutes. When compression of the radial artery is repeated within approximately 1 minute, a type C pattern is often transformed into a type B pattern, suggesting recruitment of collaterals induced by relative ischemia of the hand. Collateral development has been shown to occur in time on Doppler ultrasound examination one year after radial artery excision for bypass surgery. This phenomenon cannot easily be assessed with the modified Allen test. In type D, pulsatile blood flow and oximetry are abolished by compression of the radial artery and do not reappear within 2 minutes. As pulsatile blood flow has been correlated with healing and the absence of ischemic necrosis, the type D regimen has been considered unsuitable for the transradial approach[62].

3.   Usefulness of Allen tests and derivatives

Although ischemia is a rare complication of arterial puncture, many healthcare providers perform neither the Allen test nor the modified Allen test before accessing the radial artery, as there is conflicting evidence on the accuracy of this test for assessing ulnar artery patency or adequacy of collateral circulation. A study published in 2007 by Kohonen et al[64], carried out between October 2000 and April 2005, enrolled 145 patients. Subjects were selected for coronary artery bypass grafting, with possible use of the radial artery as a graft. Emergency cases and patients over 60 years of age were excluded. The mean age was 52.0 years. Male gender predominated (130 vs. 15) and most patients were right-handed (136 vs. 9). Patients underwent the Allen test, Doppler ultrasound and digital plethysmography. All tests were performed by the same medical examiner in the clinical physiology laboratory. The non-dominant arm was studied and, if there was a contraindication to radial artery harvesting, the dominant arm was also tested. Only non-dominant arms were included in this study. Most patients had a positive Allen test, but 23% were negative (abnormal). Ultrasound revealed anatomical abnormalities in 10 patients and circulatory deficits in 17. Thirteen patients had both circulatory and anatomical abnormalities. The sensitivity of the Allen test was 73.2% and specificity 97.1%, making it a good screening test for hand circulation prior to radial artery harvesting for coronary artery bypass grafting.Numerous other studies, including those by Ruengsakulrach et al. in 2001[65] and Agarwal et al. in 2020[66] have demonstrated that modified Allen tests are valid for screening for collateral circulation in the hand.In the RADAR study (Should Intervention Through Radial Approach be Denied to Patients With Negative Allen's Test Results?)[67], a prospective, single-center study conducted between October 2007 and June 2009, designed to assess the safety and feasibility of the catheterization and transradial intervention in patients with abnormal or intermediate Allen test results compared with those with normal results; Valgimigli et al[67] studied the relationship between functional assessment of the double vascularity of the hand (using the Allen test and plethysmography-oximetry) and measures of distal ischemia (lactate). Of a total of 942 patients undergoing transradial catheterization 203 were recruited, of whom 83, 60 and 60 had normal, intermediate and abnormal Allen test results, respectively (Allen test results were were defined as normal, intermediate or abnormal if maximum palmar recoloration after release of compression was achieved within 5 s, between 6 and 10 s, or after 10 s, respectively). Lactate did not differ between the 3 study groups after the procedure (1.85 ±0.93 mmol/l in patients with normal Allen test results, 1.85 ±0.66 mmol/l in those with intermediate results, and 1.97 ±0.71 mmol/l in those with abnormal results; p = 0.59) or at other points in the study (Fig. 22). Plethysmographic readings showed improvements in ulnopalmar collateralization in patients with abnormal Allen test results, suggesting increased ulnar flow after radial access. Hand strength test results and discomfort assessments did not differ between groups. No ischemic hand complications occurred. On the basis of the RADAR results, some authors believe that denial of radial access for diagnostic angiography or interventions solely on the basis of an abnormal curve of an Allen or oximetry-plethysmography test is not justified, as these tests are not scientifically predictive of a pathological increase in lactate levels, hand weakness or persistent discomfort during or after transradial catheterization. The time has come to remove this test from pre-procedural triage for transradial catheterization[68].

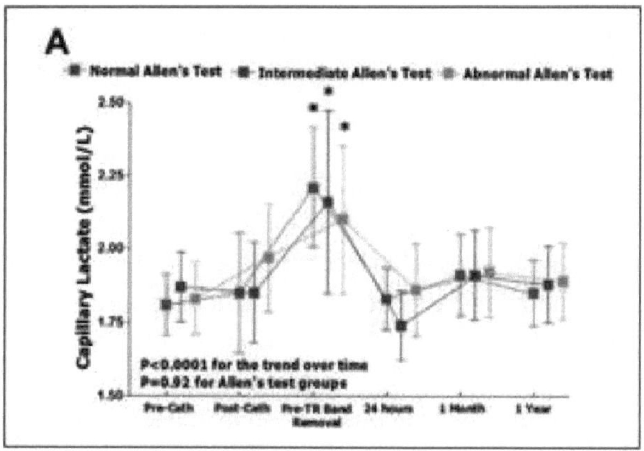


Figure 22. Thumb capillary lactate levels did not differ after compared with before catheterization (cath) independently of Allen test (AT) results obtained at baseline.[67]

In 2015, Bonnett et al examined the use of the barb test as an alternative to the modified Allen test in patients undergoing radial artery catheterization and concluded that the barb test is more sensitive and less dependent on the subjective judgment of nurses[69]. This same result was confirmed by the study of Mohamed Zarea et al in 2021[70]. In conclusion, there is no consistent evidence to support the routine use of the barb test as an alternative tool for detecting hand collateral circulation. Also on the basis of previous evidence, the use of the modified Allen test can neither be denied nor supported for predicting the risk of ischemic complications of the hand, however for medico-legal reasons it is still widely accepted and used in the USA.

## II.PATIENT SET-UP AND ARTERIAL PUNCTURE

Distal radial access can be obtained from either the right or left radial artery, assuming both are acceptable in terms of Allen's test. For some operators, the left radial is preferable, as catheter handling is similar to femoral access. The left arm is placed comfortably on a cushion above the patient, and the left hand is positioned at the patient's right groin (Figures 23 and 24). After disinfection, the patient is covered with a sterile drape containing four holes (two radial, two femoral). The left femoral hole is placed on the dorsal surface of the patient's left hand.

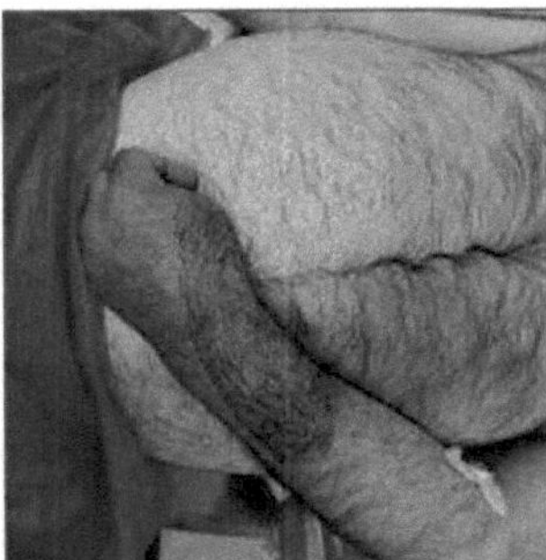

Figure 23. Installing the hand for left distal radial access

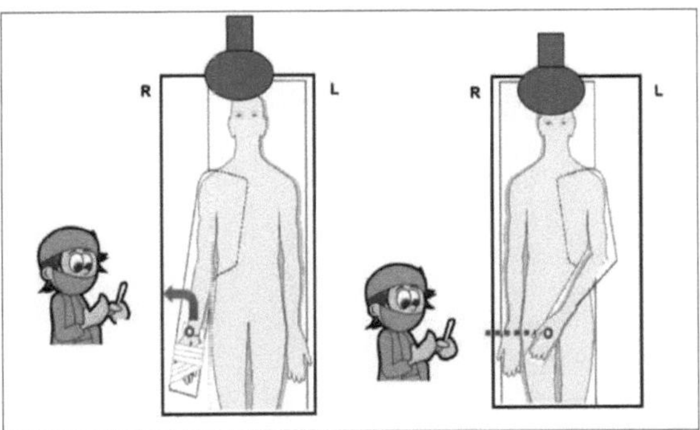


Figure 24. Patient set-up for left and right ARD1

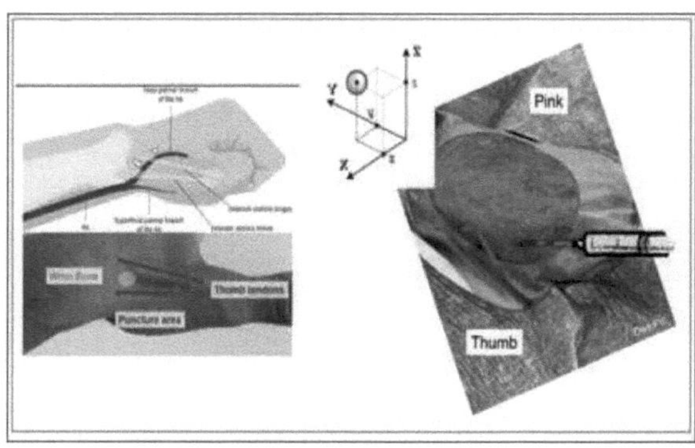


Figure 25. Anatomical snuffbox and puncture sites for ARD1

The anatomical snuffbox is a triangular-shaped space on the lateral side of the dorsal wrist, clearly visible when the thumb is extended. It is delimited by the tendons of the extensor pollicis brevis and abductor pollicis brevis on the lateral side of the wrist and the tendon of the extensor pollicis longus on the medial side. The base of the triangle is formed by the radial styloid process. The trapezoid and scaphoid bones form the lower part of the anatomical snuffbox. In this region, the radial artery is easily palpable and becomes the superior puncture site due to its superficial position and bony base (figure 25). Distal transradial access includes the snuffbox site and the very distal radial artery, which lies at the apex of the angle between the long extensor tendon of the thumb and the second metacarpal. However, most interventionalists tend to choose the snuffbox region as the site for distal radial access.

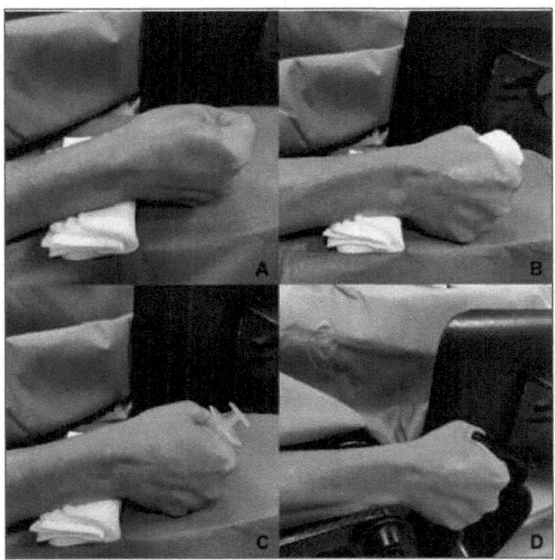

Figure 26. Installation of the right arm for puncture of the distal radial artery [71].

To expose the distal part of the radial artery at the level of the anatomical snuffbox, the patient is asked to place his thumb under the other four fingers or hold a roll of gauze, a 20 ml syringe or the handle of a system[71](figure 26). The operator positions himself close to the patient's head for the subcutaneous injection of 3 to 5 cc of xylocaine into the radial fossa, then the artery is punctured, preferably with a 21-gauge needle, at an angle of 30-45 degrees from lateral to medial.

The puncture needle is aimed at the strongest pulse point, proximal to the snuffbox. anatomical.A transfixing puncture is not recommended, as the needle contact with the periosteum of the scaphoid bone or trapezium can be painful, which can encourage spasm.After successful puncture, a small-gauge 0.21" J-guide is inserted, followed by a desilet with introducer. The creation of a buttonhole can assist the passage of the desilet (figure 27).

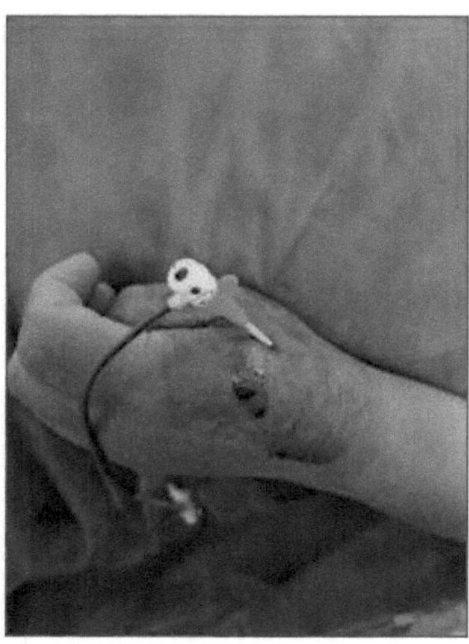

Figure 27. Stent in place after distal radial puncture

After administration of a cocktail   spasmolytic cocktail (200mcg nitroglycerin and 5mg verapamil) and a bolus of heparin[15], the operator can take up position at the patient's knee to manipulate the 0.035" J guide, catheters and intracoronary devices. In a publication appearing in "The British Journal of Cardiology" in 2021, Lim et al[72] reported on a patient admitted for preoperative coronary angiography of a stenosis aortic stenosis stenosis at who coronary angiography was performed via a 4 Fr right distal radial access without administration of heparin. The procedure was uncomplicated. The rationale for this attitude, which runs counter to current conventions in this field, is as follows that distal puncture has a very low rate of occlusion of the radial artery, enabling them to avoid using heparin, and that this, together with the use of a 4Fr catheter, enables rapid and effective hemostasis with low compression, thus "killing two birds with one stone". This attitude has not been validated and requires further investigation.

# III. HEMOSTASE

After the procedure, haemostasis can be easily achieved after removal of the mesh, using a haemostasis device adapted to the distal radial or a gauze pad wrapped in an elastic bandage and left in place for two to three hours[15](figure 28).

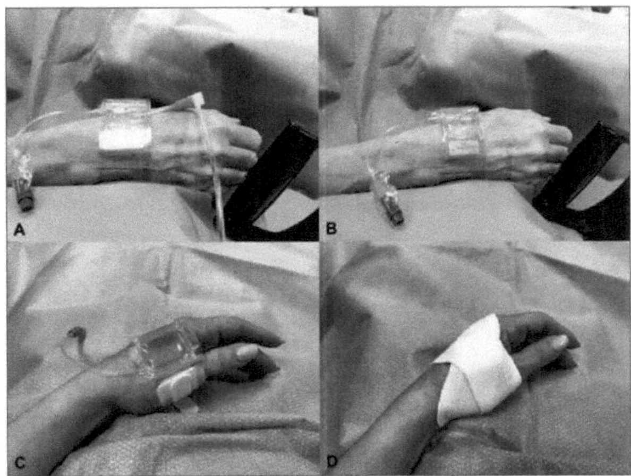

Figure 28. Dedicated hemostasis device for the distal radial [71].

# IV. THE ROLE OF DOPPLER IN APPROACH SELECTION :

Palpation is not a reliable method, as the radial artery's small caliber is close to the limit of digital discrimination between 2 points, which is 2 to 4 mm, hence the difficulty of locating it accurately using this technique. It may also be hypoplastic, calcified, mobile, collapsed, or associated with other anatomical anomalies or a dilated radial vein. In addition, the distal radial artery may be collateralized, and its pulse can be palpated even in the presence of an upstream occlusion. All these difficulties can delay access to the radial artery in the event of catheterization, and may contribute to the reluctance of the operator to adopt this route, particularly in the case of primary angioplasty. 4 years after the advent of DRA, Kiemeneij et al, published a follow-up review arguing for the inclusion of ultrasound in the stages of this technique[73]. Ultrasound allows identification of anatomical landmarks and precise access to the vessel. The authors strongly encourage the use of ultrasound, particularly at the beginning of the DRA learning curve. Installation requires no special equipment or preparation. In addition to the standard equipment required for radial artery cannulation, operators need :

• A high-frequency ultrasound device (e.g. 5 to 10 MHz or more),
• A linear probe, sterile water-based lubricant in a single-use sachet (preferable to a bottle of multi-use ultrasound gel),
• A sterile probe cover to cover the probe and probe cable.

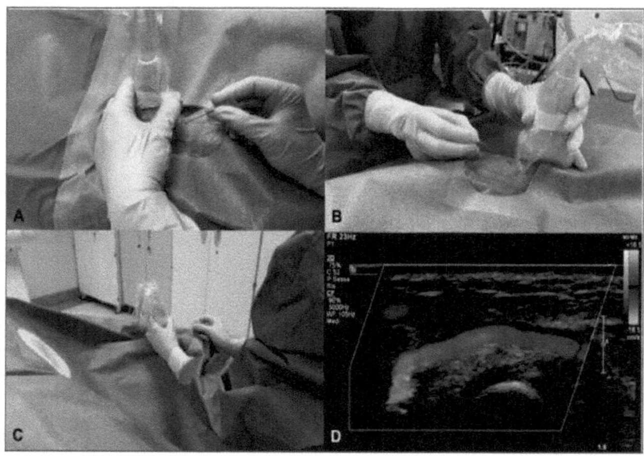

Figure 29. Distal radial puncture under ultrasound guidance [71].

The probe is placed on the wrist at the level of the anatomical snuffbox (figure 29). Vessel visualization can be enhanced by setting the ultrasound depth to the minimum and adjusting the gain. The examiner's hand should rest partially on the patient, and only light pressure should be exerted on the soft tissues. Vigorous pressure from the transducer compresses the artery. The artery is visualized as an anechoic or dark circle, which can be distinguished from the veins by the pulsation of the vessel. Manual compression, pulsed Doppler and color Doppler are additional tools that facilitate artery detection. The transverse ultrasound view (short axis, cross-section) is easy to obtain and is the best for identifying veins and arteries and their orientation in relation to each other (figure 30). The long-axis ultrasound view is technically more difficult to obtain, but the entire needle is imaged continuously, guaranteeing precise intraluminal placement. In the early stages of using ultrasound tracking, a learning curve is to be expected, but this should not deter operators from using this valuable know-how. Basic expertise in ARC is necessary before moving on to ARD, but no prior ultrasound experience is required. A common misconception is that once the needle has pierced the skin, there's no point in inspecting the wrist. Instead, the operator should look at the ultrasound screen and move the probe to find the needle tip. The main anatomical structures to be identified in the anatomical snuffbox are illustrated in figure 30.

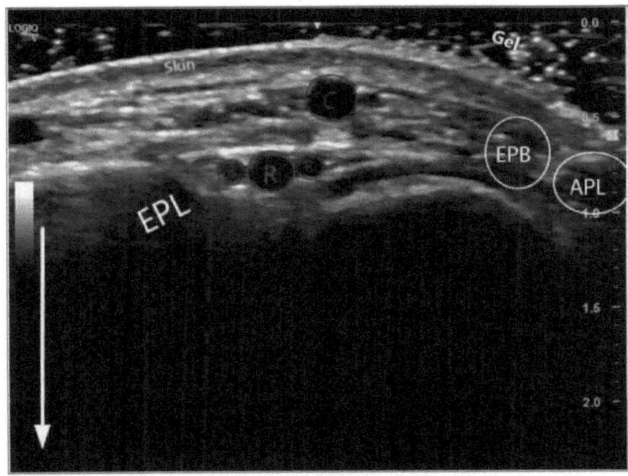

Figure 30. Transverse ultrasound image at the level of the anatomical snuffbox. On the surface, the cephalic vein (C), in depth, the radial artery (R red) accompanied by 2 radial veins (R blue). The snuffbox is surrounded by the extensor pollicis longus (EPL), extensor pollicis brevis (EPB), abductor pollicis longus (APL) and scaphoid (S)[74].

The radial artery must be scanned along the snuffbox in short-axis view, then in long-axis view in order to select the best puncture site, aiming for sufficient caliber (ideally> 1.8 mm) and the absence of tortuosity and disease (figure 31).

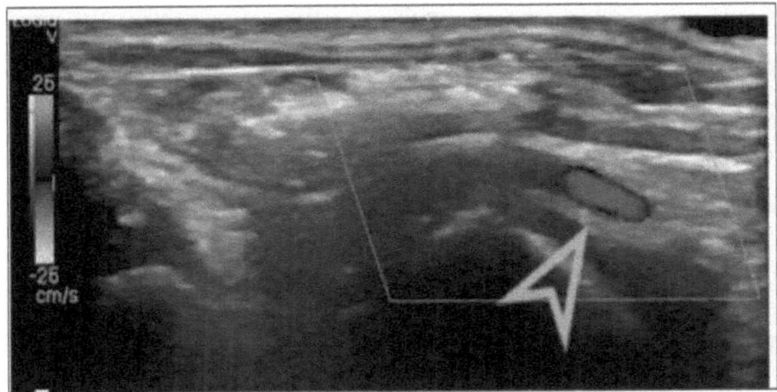

Figure 31. Normal radial artery [74]

The puncture zone (the triangle) is bisected by the tendon of the extensor pollicis longus muscle, which is prominent and easily palpated. The true area of the snuffbox is proximal to the extensor pollicis longus tendon, as illustrated in figure 32 (blue arrow), where the artery is located lateral to the tendon.

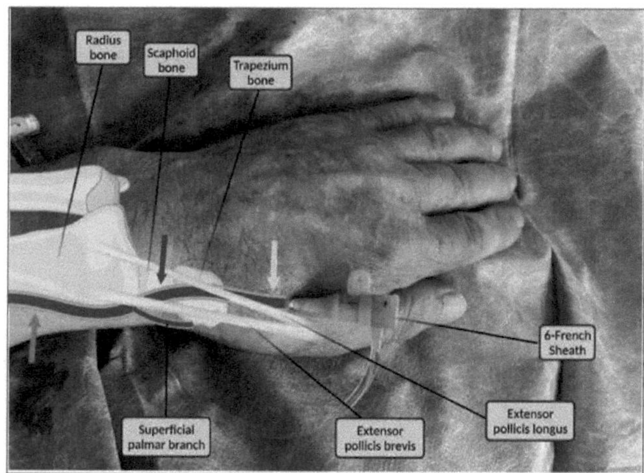


*Figure 32.* Structures of the anatomical snuffbox in relation to the arterial sheath. Common radial puncture sites: proximal (green arrow), anatomical snuffbox (blue arrow) and distal dorsal (yellow arrow). [74]

The artery then continues under the tendon, entering the first intermetacarpal space, where it can be palpated and punctured again (region on the back of the hand, which is not the preference of operators (figure 32, yellow arrow), and finally, it continues its course medially and deeply, forming anastomoses with the ulnar artery. The skin is then punctured parallel to the probe, at its exact center. As the artery is very superficial, immediately under the skin, even a small haematoma can compress it, making subsequent attempts more difficult. The vessel can be punctured as long as the blood flow is visible on the Doppler [74]. No palpation of the artery is required, and the operator looks at the ultrasound screen. The needle can be tilted by more than 45 degrees. In some cases, the guide may encounter resistance due to tortuosity; leaving the needle free rather than fixing it with the hand can help overcome acute angles, sometimes a 0.014″ coronary guide is used[74].

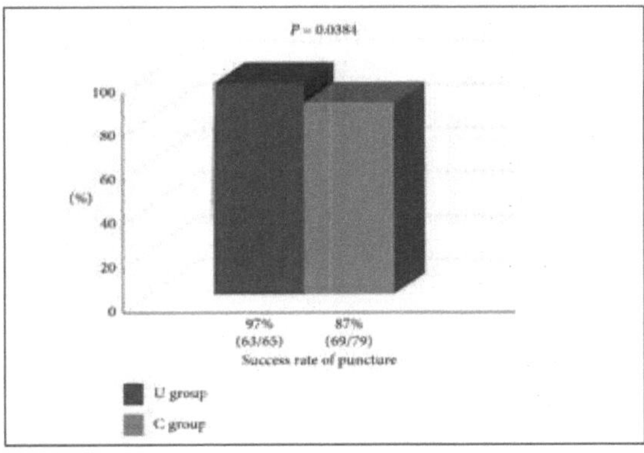


Figure 33. Puncture success rate [75].C(conventional
conventional)U(ultrasound-guided puncture).

In the only study comparing ultrasound-guided DRA with palpation-guided
DRA, ultrasound guidance increased the DRA success rate from 87 % to
97%[75] (Fig. 33). Also positive signals come from another trial, more relevant
because it studied hand function after DRA, showing no impairment, and where
the operators made extensive use of ultrasound (85%)[76]. A further role for
ultrasound in assisting DRA was demonstrated in a recent pilot study in which
chronic radial artery occlusion was retrogradely recanalized in 30 patients,
accessing the distal part of the artery by ultrasound, in the only segment where it
remained permeable (by collateralization). The anterograde damped Doppler
sign or reversed flow through the palmar arch were positive signs that puncture
could be performed at this level, even if the pulse was not palpable[77] (figures
34 and 35).

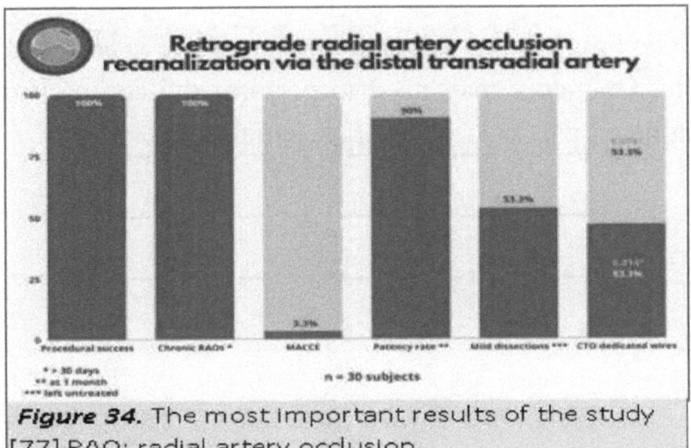


**Figure 34.** The most important results of the study
[77].RAO: radial artery occlusion.

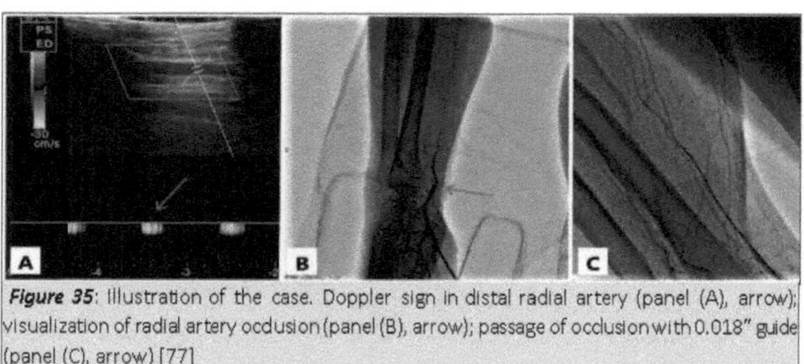

Figure 35: Illustration of the case. Doppler sign in distal radial artery (panel (A), arrow); visualization of radial artery occlusion (panel (B), arrow); passage of occlusion with 0.018" guide (panel (C), arrow) [77]

Clinical imaging is safe, cost-effective, easy to learn and safe to use,

## V. TECHNICAL LIMITS

The limitations of the distal transradial approach are similar to those of all radial artery accesses, including:

- Radial artery tortuosity,
- Anatomical variations,
- Tortuosities of the subclavian.

In addition, and as with any new procedure, there is a learning curve for the distal radial approach. Puncture of the distal radial can be difficult and time-consuming due to its smaller diameter. Women have a smaller diameter and a higher rate of puncture failure than men. Also, the small-caliber distal radial artery can limit the size of introducers and catheters used. This can affect the success of highly complex procedures. In selected patients, the use of a 7 Fr sheath is feasible and safe[78].Another problem is catheter length. Most catheters are currently designed for a conventional puncture site, so these devices may not be long enough when the puncture site is around 5 cm from the conventional site. Operators may need to perform the coronary procedure "on the tip" of the catheter, particularly in larger patients.

## VI. LEARNING CURVE

Despite the feasibility and potential benefits of DRA, interventional
cardiologists are still finding it difficult to implement this new vascular
approach, due to the lack of data concerning the learning curve, in which the
operator's skills gradually improve with experience, and the choice of patients
for initiation of DRA. Although the success rate of DRA has been analyzed in
several studies, there are no data on the number of cases that need to be
performed to achieve a consistently high success rate.

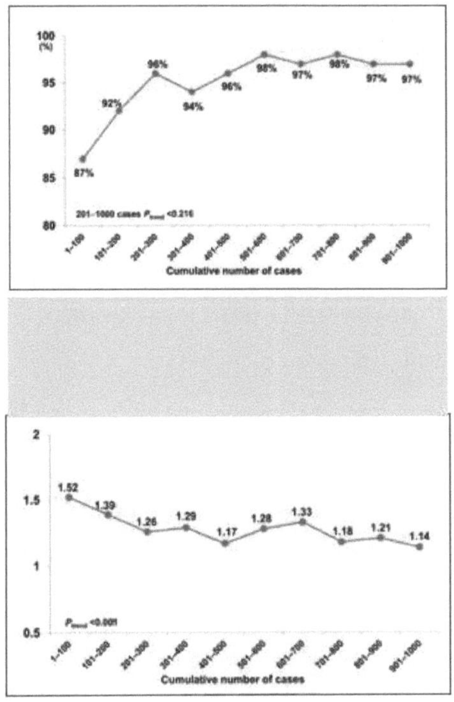

Figure 37. Time trend in success rate of distal radial access showing stable
success rate (> 94%) after200 cases[79].

Figure 36. Time trend in distal radial access puncture attempts showing a
significant decrease from 1.52 per 1-100 patients to 1.14 per 901-. 1000 patients.
[79]

Roh et al[79] in a study designed to investigate the learning curve for performing coronary angiography and angioplasty via DRA, and also to analyze factors leading to failure of this approach, retrospectively analyzed data from 1000 patients who underwent coronary angiography and angioplasty via DRA by a single experienced radial operator. The primary endpoint was the DRA success rate per 100 cases. In addition, predictors of DRA failure were analyzed. A total of 952 (95.2%) of the 1,000 patients underwent successful DRA. After the 200-case experiment, the DRA success rate was maintained at over 94% (Figure 36), and there was no difference in the success rate per 100 cases ($P_{trend}$ = 0.216).Factors predictive of failure were female gender [odds ratio (OR) 1.84, 95% confidence interval (CI) 1.01-3.39, P = 0.049] and a systolic blood pressure (SBP) of < 120 mm (OR 1.87, 95% CI 1.04-3.36,P = 0,036). The mean number of puncture attempts was 1.27 ± 0.61 for all patients successfully completing DRA. Puncture attempts decreased progressively from 1.52 to 1.14 (P < 0.001) (figure 37). The median duration of ARD was 117.5 [81.0-203.3] s. In addition, the duration of DRA decreased progressively when analyzing the trend per 100 patients (P < 0.001). (Figure 38)

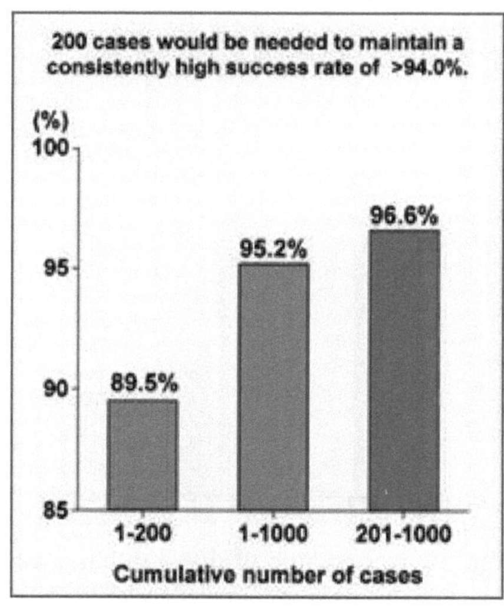


Figure 38. DRA success rate on a total of 1000 patients [79].

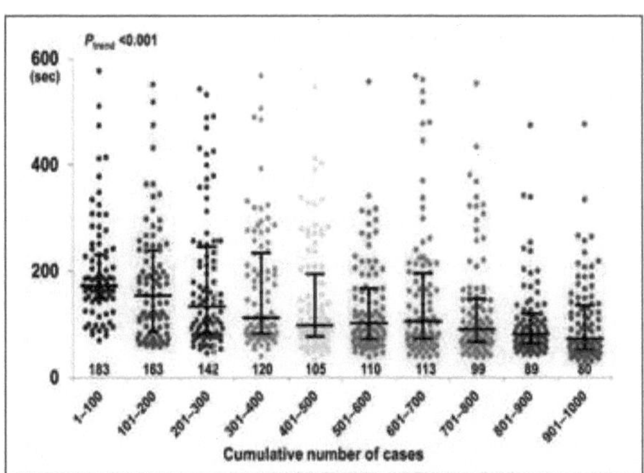


Figure 39. Trend analysis of median distal radial access time showing a significant decrease from 183 s for 1-100 patients to 80 s for 901-1000 patients. [79]

In this study, the authors show us that a learning curve of at least 200 procedures would be required to obtain a stable DRA with a success rate > 94% (figure 39). Moreover, this new approach could fail in women and patients with low PAS.

# COMPLICATIONS

As expected, DRA for cardiac procedures offers superior safety and satisfaction[80]. As a new approach to cardiac catheterization, access-related complications must also be taken into account by operators, such as OAR, radial spasm, bleeding and hematoma, and injury to the superficial branch of the radial nerve.

## I. RADIAL ARTERY OCCLUSION

Stenosis or occlusion after catheterization via the ATR will affect the future use of the radial artery, which becomes one of the important reasons for interventionists to find alternative approaches. Post-catheterization stenosis and occlusion of the radial artery are common and linked to several factors, including[81] :

- The female sex,
- Age,
- Manual compression
- And the diameter of the radial artery.

Wakeyama et al[82] found radial artery hypertrophy by intravascular ultrasound (IVUS) after transradial intervention.

After 6 months, intima-media volume in patients who underwent transradial artery intervention increased significantly, while lumen volume and vessel volume decreased significantly. Recently, post-catheterization disorders of the radial artery, including intimal dissection, medial calcification, intimal lesion, medial hypertrophy and adventitial neovascularization, have been observed by optical coherence tomography at different time periods[38]. The incidence of distal radial artery occlusion is relatively low in recent literature, ranging from 0.0 to 5.2%. In one large retrospective study, the incidence of distal radial artery occlusion was only 0.61% (10/1661) [39]. In another large retrospective study carried out in the Russian Federation, the total rate of OAR was 2.2% (22/1009) in the anatomical snuffbox approach [38]. The distribution of occlusion sites was 0.1% in the forearm radial artery, 1.8% in the anatomical snuffbox and 0.3% in both the forearm radial artery and the snuffbox. The occlusion rate in the forearm radial artery by DRA was reduced by 90% compared with that obtained by CRA (0.4% vs. 4.2%). However, the occlusion rate was reported to be around 5% in a randomized study involving a sample of 100 people[41].In another recent study, Horák et al[83] assessed proximal and distal radial artery patency after coronary procedures performed via the distal radial artery. Ultrasonography, the most reliable method, was used to diagnose radial artery occlusions. 115 patients undergoing catheterization via the distal radial access were evaluated.

After the procedure and successful hemostasis (80 ± 36 min), arterial patency and diameter at the conventional transradial access and distal puncture sites (either in the anatomical snuffbox or in the dorsal distal radial) were assessed. No radial occlusions were found either proximally or distally, and there were no other complications. significant. The mean diameter of the radial artery at the conventional puncture site was 2.86 ± 0.49 mm and at the distal puncture site 2.31± 0.47 mm (p< 0.001). Post-procedural compression time of the distal radial artery was very short (Fig. 40).

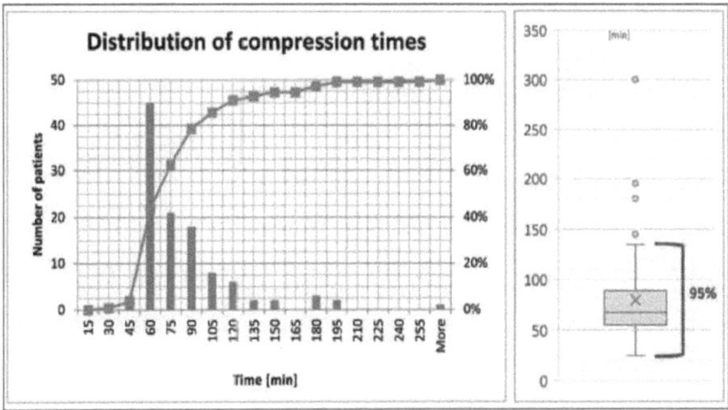


Figure 40: Compression time: cumulative histogram and box plot.

The box plot (right-hand side of figure) shows that around 80% of patients had compression times of less than 90 minutes, and almost 95% of patients had compression times of less than 135 minutes. [83] The low occlusion rate in ARD can be explained by the following reasons:

• The artery at the snuffbox is small and superficial, with a bony platform underneath. Hemostasis does not require excessive pressure from the compression device or bandage.
• What's more, compression time is much shorter with ARD than with ARC.
• The hemostatic device is limited to compressing the vessel.
• During hemostasis, anterograde flow through the superficial palmar arch can be maintained even after occlusion of the distal radial artery, thus reducing the risk of retrograde thrombosis.

• Intermittent compression of the ipsilateral ulnar artery after pulling the DRA sheath to promote anterograde flow into the radial artery can minimize the risk of radial artery occlusion[84].

Of particular note is the fact that the rate of radial artery occlusion may increase with time after surgery. Researchers have found that the occlusion rate may increase slightly one month after surgery compared with 24 hours after surgery, which may be associated with remodelling of the vessel[78], [85].

## II. BLEEDING, HEMATOMA AND PSEUDO-ANEURYSM

Due to the structure of the snuffbox, with a bony base surrounded by tendons, the incidence of severe bleeding, pseudoaneurysms and hematomas is infrequent. Whether using a hemostatic device or a bandage, hemostasis in the region of the distal radial artery is easier and quicker than in the forearm, which can reduce the length of hospital stay and the nurses' daily workload. In patients undergoing coronary angiography, hemostasis can be achieved by compressing the puncture site with the finger for 15 minutes. Even in the case of angioplasty, digital pressure can achieve hemostasis in patients with an ACT < 250 s at the end of the procedure[84]. Although minor hematomas sometimes occur, the prevalence of major hematoma is actually very low. The prevalence of hematomas larger than 10 cm was reported to be only 0.2% in a large retrospective study[38]. The hematoma was probably precipitated by[85] :

• Incorrect compression position,
• The use of two antiplatelet agents and heparin,
• Advanced age,
• Fragile skin
• Multiple puncture attempts.

Pseudoaneurysm is extremely rare. In 2019, Prejean et al [86] reported a case of pseudoaneurysm in the distal left radial artery occurring 20 h after introducer removal (figure 41), which was successfully treated with a further 12-h compression (figure42).

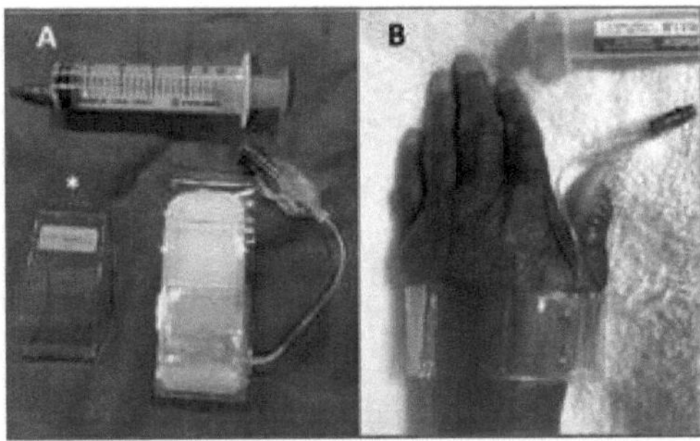

Figure 41. Management of pseudoaneurysm of the left distal radial artery by compression [86]

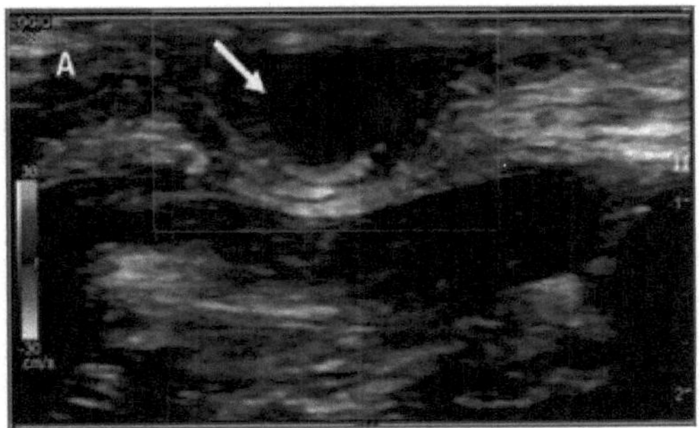

Figure 42. Vascular ultrasound of the distal left radial artery. A 2.3 × 1.5 × 1.7 cm pseudoaneurysm of the distal left radial artery with partial thrombosis (white arrow) is observed. [86]

## III. NUMBNESS

Theoretically, the space of the anatomical snuffbox is narrow, and the superficial branch of the radial nerve is close to the radial artery. Repeated punctures in this space and long duration of compression can damage the superficial branch of the radial nerve, leading to numbness of the fingers. In a prospective real-life observational study, Lee et al[85] reported 2 cases out of 141 (1.4%) with numbness. Finger numbness in 2 cases (1.0%) was also observed in a multicenter Japanese study[44]. Ultrasound-guided puncture may increase the success rate and reduce the number of puncture attempts, potentially reducing the incidence of this complication.

# IV. PAIN

During the ATR, the hand is placed in a supinated position during the operation, causing discomfort for the patient. This is particularly true when working on the left hand and when the patient is obese. Also, the blockage of blood flow during compression can lead to significant hand swelling and pain, which can reduce patient satisfaction with the procedure. These situations are naturally absent with distal access, as the hand is placed in a natural position during the procedure, and in addition, due to the special anatomical structure, compression after catheter removal need not completely block blood flow, and the hemostatic time is relatively short. This obviously increases patient satisfaction. In a case-control study, researchers studied patient satisfaction and found that the satisfaction rate in the ARD group was 89%, which was slightly higher than in the ATR group (87%)[36].

# CONCLUSION

The use of the distal radial approach is a promising technique in interventional cardiology, offering multiple advantages over the conventional radial approach, the most important of which is to reduce the risk of radial artery occlusion, offer greater comfort for both patient and operator during procedures requiring a left vascular approach, and reduce the time needed to achieve hemostasis. Although further research is needed to include it in recommendations or to make it a reference technique, its use is set to become widespread in interventional cardiology centers.

**BIBLIOGRAPHY**

[1] A. Bajaj, S. Pancholy, A. Sothwal, Y. Nawaz, and P. Boruah, "Transradial Versus Transfemoral Access for Percutaneous Coronary Intervention of Unprotected Left Main Coronary Artery Stenosis: A Systematic Review and Meta-Analysis," Cardiovascular Revascularization Medicine, vol. 20, no. 9, pp. 790-798, Sept. 2019, doi: 10.1016/j.carrev.2018.10.025.

[2] G. Ferrante et al, "Radial Versus Femoral Access for Coronary Interventions Across the Entire Spectrum of Patients With Coronary Artery Disease," JACC: Cardiovascular Interventions, vol. 9, no. 14, pp. 1419-1434, Jul. 2016, doi: 10.1016/j.jcin.2016.04.014.

[3] M. Valgimigli et al, "Radial versus femoral access and bivalirudin versus unfractionated heparin in invasively managed patients with acute coronary syndrome (MATRIX): final 1-year results of a multicentre, randomised controlled trial", The Lancet, vol. 392, no. 10150, pp. 835-848, Sept. 2018, doi: 10.1016/S0140-6736(18)31714-8.

[4] A. P. Banning et al, "The Task Force on myocardial revascularization of the European Society of Cardiology (ESC) and European Association for Cardio-Thoracic Surgery (EACTS)", Thoracic Surgery, 2018.

[5] J. S. Lawton et al, "2021 ACC/AHA/SCAI Guideline for Coronary Artery Revascularization: Executive Summary: A Report of the American College of Cardiology/American Heart Association Joint Committee on Clinical Practice Guidelines", Circulation, vol. 145, no. 3, Jan. 2022, doi: 10.1161/CIR.0000000000001039.

[6] S. Radner, "Thoracal Aortography by Catheterization from the Radlal Artery", Acta Radiologica, vol. 29, no. 2, pp. 178-180, Jan. 1948, doi: 10.3109/00016924809132437.

[7] L. Campeau, "Percutaneous radial artery approach for coronary angiography," Cathet. Cardiovasc. Diagn. vol. 16, no. 1, pp. 3-7, Jan. 1989, doi: 10.1002/ccd.1810160103.

[8] F. Kiemeneij and G. Jan Laarman, "Percutaneous transradial artery approach for coronary stent implantation", Cathet. Cardiovasc. Diagn. vol. 30, no. 2, pp. 173-178, Oct. 1993, doi: 10.1002/ccd.1810300220.

[9] A. A. Kolkailah, R. S. Alreshq, A. M. Muhammed, M. E. Zahran, M. Anas El-Wegoud, and A. F. Nabhan, "Transradial versus transfemoral approach for diagnostic coronary angiography and percutaneous coronary intervention in

people with coronary artery disease," Cochrane Database of Systematic Reviews, vol. 2018, no. 4, Apr. 2018, doi: 10.1002/14651858.CD012318.pub2.

[10]J. Aoun, L. Hattar, K. Dgayli, G. Wong, and T. Bhat, "Update on complications and their management during transradial cardiac catheterization," Expert Review of Cardiovascular Therapy, vol. 17, no. 10, pp. 741-751, Oct. 2019, doi: 10.1080/14779072.2019.1675510.

[11]M. Rashid et al, "Radial Artery Occlusion After Transradial Interventions: A Systematic Review and Meta-Analysis", JAHA, vol. 5, no. 1, p. e002686, Jan. 2016, doi: 10.1161/JAHA.115.002686.

[12]J. J. Amato, E. Solod, and R. J. Cleveland, "A 'second' radial artery for monitoring the perioperative pediatric cardiac patient," Journal of Pediatric Surgery, vol. 12, no. 5, pp. 715-717, Oct. 1977, doi: 10.1016/0022-3468(77)90399-2.

[13]A. Babunashvili and D. Dundua, "Recanalization and reuse of early occluded radial artery within 6 days after previous transradial diagnostic procedure," Cathet. Cardiovasc. Intervent, vol. 77, no. 4, pp. 530-536, March 2011, doi: 10.1002/ccd.22846.

[14]"Roghani-Dehkordi F. Merits of more distal accesses in the hand for coronary angiography and intervention. Proceedings of the 4th International Cardiovascular Joint Congress in Isfahan; 2016 Nov. 24-25; Isfahan, Iran".

[15]F. Kiemeneij, "Left distal transradial access in the anatomical snuffbox for coronary angiography (ldTRA) and interventions (ldTRI)," EuroIntervention, vol. 13, no. 7, pp. 851-857, Sept. 2017, doi: 10.4244/EIJ-D-17-00079.

[16]G. A. Sgueglia, A. Di Giorgio, A. Gaspardone, and A. Babunashvili, "Anatomic Basis and Physiological Rationale of Distal Radial Artery Access for Percutaneous Coronary and Endovascular Procedures," JACC: Cardiovascular Interventions, vol. 11, no. 20, pp. 2113-2119, Oct. 2018, doi: 10.1016/j.jcin.2018.04.045.

[17]A. Aminian et al, "Distal Versus Conventional Radial Access for Coronary Angiography and Intervention," JACC: Cardiovascular Interventions, vol. 15, no. 12, pp. 1191-1201, June 2022, doi: 10.1016/j.jcin.2022.04.032.

[18] N. Gocmen, H. Selim, M. Edizer, and O. Magde, "Importance of Anatomical Landmarks on Axillary Neurovascular Territories for Surgery," in Current Concepts in Plastic Surgery, F. Agullo, Ed., InTech, 2012. doi: 10.5772/28367.

[19] Drake, R., Vogl, A. and Mitchell, A., Gray's Anatomy for Students, 3 rd edition. London: Churchill Livingston Elsevier, 2014.

[20] Gray, Henry. Anatomy of the Human Body. Philadelphia: Lea & Febiger, 1918; Bartleby.com, 2000. www.bartleby.com/107/.

[21] B.-S. Yoo et al, "Anatomical consideration of the radial artery for transradial coronary procedures: arterial diameter, branching anomaly and vessel tortuosity", International Journal of Cardiology, vol. 101, no. 3, pp. 421-427, June 2005, doi: 10.1016/j.ijcard.2004.03.061.

[22] H. Shima, K. Ohno, K. Michi, K. Egawa, and R. Takiguchi, "An anatomical study on the forearm vascular system," Journal of Cranio-Maxillofacial Surgery, vol. 24, no. 5, pp. 293-299, Oct. 1996, doi: 10.1016/S1010-5182(96)80062-X.

[23] S. Nagai et al, "Ultrasonic assessment of vascular complications in coronary angiography and angioplasty after transradial approach", The American Journal of Cardiology, vol. 83, no. 2, pp. 180-186, Jan. 1999, doi: 10.1016/S0002-9149(98)00821-2.

[24] R. Haładaj, G. Wysiadecki, Z. Dudkiewicz, M. Polguj, and M. Topol, "The High Origin of the Radial Artery (Brachioradial Artery): Its Anatomical Variations, Clinical Significance, and Contribution to the Blood Supply of the Hand," BioMed Research International, vol. 2018, pp. 1-11, June 2018, doi: 10.1155/2018/1520929.

[25]K. H. Narsinh et al, "Radial artery access anatomy: considerations for neuroendovascular procedures", J NeuroIntervent Surg, vol. 13, no. 12, pp. 1139-1144, Dec. 2021, doi: 10.1136/neurintsurg-2021-017871.

[26]R. H. Dossani et al, "Endovascular management of radial artery loop for neuroangiography: Case series", Interv Neuroradiol, vol. 27, no. 4, pp. 566-570, August 2021, doi: 10.1177/15910199920982812.

[27]G. Wysiadecki, M. Polguj, R. Haładaj, and M. Topol, "Low origin of the radial artery: a case study including a review of literature and proposal of an embryological explanation," Anat Sci Int, vol. 92, no. 2, pp. 293-298, March 2017, doi: 10.1007/s12565-016-0371-9.

[28]M. Rodríguez-Niedenführ, T. Vázquez, I. G. Parkin, and J. R. Sañudo, "Arterial patterns of the human upper limb: update of anatomical variations and embryological development".

[29]R. E. S. Tan and A. Lahiri, "Vascular Anatomy of the Hand in Relation to

Flaps," Hand Clinics, vol. 36, no. 1, pp. 1-8, Feb. 2020, doi: 10.1016/j.hcl.2019.08.001.

[30]"Jaschtschinski S. Morphologie und Topologie des Arcus volaris sublimes und profundus des Menschen. Anat Heft 1897;7:161- 88".

[31]G. A. Sgueglia, A. Di Giorgio, A. Gaspardone, and A. Babunashvili, "Anatomic Basis and Physiological Rationale of Distal Radial Artery Access for Percutaneous Coronary and Endovascular Procedures," JACC: Cardiovascular Interventions, vol. 11, no. 20, pp. 2113-2119, Oct. 2018, doi: 10.1016/j.jcin.2018.04.045.

[32]G. Cai, H. Huang, F. Li, G. Shi, X. Yu, and L. Yu, "Distal transradial access: a review of the feasibility and safety in cardiovascular angiography and intervention", BMC Cardiovasc Disord, vol. 20, no. 1, p. 356, Dec. 2020, doi: 10.1186/s12872-020-01625-8.

[33]S.-H. Lee, J.-W. Lee, J. W. Son, and S. W. Park, "CRT-100.93 The Procedural Success and Complication Rate of the Left Distal Transradial Approach," JACC: Cardiovascular Interventions, vol. 11, no. 4, p. S27, Feb. 2018, doi: 10.1016/j.jcin.2018.01.083.

[34]E. Soydan, "Coronary angiography using the left distal radial approach - An alternative site to conventional radial coronary angiography," Anatol J Cardiol, 2018, doi: 10.14744/AnatolJCardiol.2018.59932.

[35]Y. Kim et al, "Feasibility of Coronary Angiography and Percutaneous Coronary Intervention via Left Snuffbox Approach," Korean Circ J, vol. 48, no. 12, p. 1120, 2018, doi: 10.4070/kcj.2018.0181.

[36]S. Aoi et al, "Distal transradial artery access in the anatomical snuffbox for coronary angiography as an alternative access site for faster hemostasis," Catheter Cardiovasc Interv, vol. 94, no. 5, pp. 651-657, Nov. 2019, doi: 10.1002/ccd.28155.

[37] A. Aminian et al, "Distal Versus Conventional Radial Access for Coronary Angiography and Intervention," JACC: Cardiovascular Interventions, vol. 15, no. 12, pp. 1191-1201, June 2022, doi: 10.1016/j.jcin.2022.04.032.

[38] Kaledin, Aleksandr & Kochanov, In & Podmetin, Ps & Seletsky, Ss & Ardeev, Vn., "Distal radial artery in endovascular interventions.", 2017, doi: 10.13140/RG.2.2.13406.33600.

[39] Babunashvili A., "Novel distal transradial approach for coronary and peripheral interventions," J Am Coll Cardiol. vol. 72(13 Supplement):B323.,

2018, doi: https://doi.org/10.1016/j.jacc.2018.08.2046.

[40] W. Li et al, "Comparison of the feasibility and safety between distal transradial access and conventional transradial access in patients with acute chest pain: a single-center cohort study using propensity score matching", BMC Geriatr, vol. 23, no. 1, p. 348, June 2023, doi: 10.1186/s12877-023-04058-y.

[41] M. Koutouzis et al, "Distal Versus Traditional Radial Approach for Coronary Angiography," Cardiovascular Revascularization Medicine, vol. 20, no. 8, pp. 678-680, August 2019, doi: 10.1016/j.carrev.2018.09.018.

[42] G. Eid-Lidt, A. Rivera Rodríguez, J. Jimenez Castellanos, J. I. Farjat Pasos, K. E. Estrada López, and J. Gaspar, "Distal Radial Artery Approach to Prevent Radial Artery Occlusion Trial," JACC: Cardiovascular Interventions, vol. 14, no. 4, pp. 378-385, Feb. 2021, doi: 10.1016/j.jcin.2020.10.013.

[43] A. Achim et al, "Distal Radial Artery Access for Coronary and Peripheral Procedures: A Multicenter Experience," JCM, vol. 10, no. 24, p. 5974, Dec. 2021, doi: 10.3390/jcm10245974.

[44] Y. Mizuguchi et al, "Efficacy and safety of the distal transradial approach in coronary angiography and percutaneous coronary intervention: a Japanese multicenter experience," Cardiovasc Interv and Ther, vol. 35, no. 2, pp. 162-167, Apr. 2020, doi: 10.1007/s12928-019- 00590-0.

[45] M. I. Sanhoury, M. A. Sobhy, M. A. Saddaka, M. A. Nassar, and M. N. Elwany, "Distal radial approach between theory and clinical practice... Time to go distal!", Egypt Heart J, vol. 74, no. 1, p. 8, Dec. 2022, doi: 10.1186/s43044-022-00243-3.

[46] I. Nikolakopoulos et al, "Distal Radial Access in Chronic Total Occlusion Percutaneous Coronary Intervention: Insights From the PROGRESS-CTO Registry," J Invasive Cardiol, vol. 33, no. 9, pp. E717-E722, Sept. 2021.

[47] A. Achim et al, "Switching From Proximal to Distal Radial Artery Access for Coronary Chronic Total Occlusion Recanalization," Front. Cardiovasc. Med. vol. 9, p. 895457, May 2022, doi: 10.3389/fcvm.2022.895457.

[48] A. Achim et al, "Distal Radial Secondary Access for Transcatheter Aortic Valve Implantation: The Minimalistic Approach," Cardiovascular Revascularization Medicine, vol. 40, pp. 152-157, Jul. 2022, doi: 10.1016/j.carrev.2021.11.021.

[49]D. J. McCarthy, S. H. Chen, M.-C. Brunet, S. Shah, E. Peterson, and R. M. Starke, "Distal Radial Artery Access in the Anatomical Snuffbox for

Neurointerventions: Case Report," World Neurosurgery, vol. 122, pp. 355-359, Feb. 2019, doi: 10.1016/j.wneu.2018.11.030.

[50]F. Al Saiegh et al, "Placement of the Woven EndoBridge (WEB) device via distal transradial access in the anatomical snuffbox: A technical note", Journal of Clinical Neuroscience, vol. 69,
pp. 261-264, Nov. 2019, doi: 10.1016/j.jocn.2019.08.018.

[51]M.-C. Brunet et al, "Distal transradial access in the anatomical snuffbox for diagnostic cerebral angiography," J NeuroIntervent Surg, vol. 11, no. 7, pp. 710-713, Jul. 2019, doi: 10.1136/neurintsurg-2019-014718.

[52]P. Patel et al, "Distal Transradial Access in the Anatomic Snuffbox for Diagnostic Cerebral Angiography," AJNR Am J Neuroradiol, p. ajnr;ajnr.A6178v1, August 2019, doi: 10.3174/ajnr.A6178.

[53]S. Nardai et al, "Feasibility of distal radial access for carotid interventions: the RADCAR- DISTAL pilot study", EuroIntervention, vol. 15, no. 14, pp. 1288-1290, Feb. 2020, doi: 10.4244/EIJ-D-19-00023.
[54]G. Di Gioia et al, "Carotid Artery Stenting Using Five-French Distal Radial Vascular Access", Diagnostics, vol. 13, no. 7, p. 1266, March 2023, doi: 10.3390/diagnostics13071266.

[55]H. Hoffman et al, "Distal Transradial Access for Diagnostic Cerebral Angiography and Neurointervention: Systematic Review and Meta-analysis," AJNR Am JNeuroradiol, vol. 42, no. 5, pp. 888-895, May 2021, doi: 10.3174/ajnr.A7074.

[56]S. Maitra, B. Ray, S. Bhattacharjee, D. Baidya, D. Dhua, and R. Batra, "Distal radial arterial cannulation in adult patients: A retrospective cohort study," Saudi J Anaesth, vol. 13, no. 1, p. 60, 2019, doi: 10.4103/sja.SJA_700_18.

[57]S. Giusca, A. Schmidt, and G. Korosoglou, "A case report of distal radial puncture in a patient with acute upper limb ischaemia: the last hope of the cardiologist?", European Heart Journal - Case Reports, vol. 6, no 7, p. ytac215, Jul. 2022, doi: 10.1093/ehjcr/ytac215.

[58]U. Pua, J. Z. T. Sim, L. H. H. Quek, J. Kwan, G. H. T. Lim, and I. K. H. Huang, "Feasibility Study of "Snuffbox" Radial Access for Visceral Interventions," Journal of Vascular and Interventional Radiology, vol. 29, no. 9, pp. 1276-1280, Sept. 2018, doi: 10.1016/j.jvir.2018.05.002.

[59]A. Bartella et al, "Hand Perfusion in Patients with Physiological or

Pathological Allen's Tests," J reconstr Microsurg, vol. 35, no. 03, pp. 182-188, March 2019, doi: 10.1055/s-0038- 1668159.

[60]Allen EV. Thromboangiitis obliterans: methods of diagnosis of chronic occlusive arterial lesions distal to the wrist with illustrative cases. Am J Med Sci 1929;2:1- 8., .

[61]Zisquit J, Velasquez J, Nedeff N. Allen Test. [Updated 2022 Sep 19]. In: StatPearls [Internet]. Treasure Island (FL): StatPearls Publishing; 2023 Jan-. Available from: https://www.ncbi.nlm.nih.gov/books/NBK507816/,

[62] G. R. Barbeau, F. Arsenault, L. Dugas, S. Simard, and M. M. Larivière, "Evaluation of the ulnopalmar arterial arches with pulse oximetry and plethysmography: Comparison with the Allen's test in 1010 patients," American Heart Journal, vol. 147, no. 3, pp. 489-493, March 2004, doi: 10.1016/j.ahj.2003.10.038.

[63] J. Habib, L. Baetz, and B. Satiani, "Assessment of collateral circulation to the hand prior to radial artery harvest," Vasc Med, vol. 17, no. 5, pp. 352-361, Oct. 2012, doi: 10.1177/1358863X12451514.

[64] M. Kohonen, O. Teerenhovi, T. Terho, J. Laurikka, and M. Tarkka, "Is the Allen test reliable enough?", European Journal of Cardio-Thoracic Surgery, vol. 32, no. 6, pp. 902-905, Dec. 2007, doi: 10.1016/j.ejcts.2007.08.017.

[65] P. Ruengsakulrach, M. Brooks, D. L. Hare, I. Gordon, and B. F. Buxton, "Preoperative assessment of hand circulation by means of Doppler ultrasonography and the modified Allen test", The Journal of Thoracic and Cardiovascular Surgery, vol. 121, no. 3, pp. 526-531, March 2001, doi: 10.1067/mtc.2001.112468.

[66] T. Agarwal, V. Agarwal, P. Agarwal, S. Thakur, R. Bobba, and D. Sharma, "Assessment of collateral hand circulation by modified Allen's test in normal Indian subjects," Journal of Clinical Orthopaedics and Trauma, vol. 11, no. 4, pp. 626-629, Jul. 2020, doi: 10.1016/j.jcot.2020.04.004.

[67] M. Valgimigli, G. Campo, C. Penzo, M. Tebaldi, S. Biscaglia, and R. Ferrari, "Transradial Coronary Catheterization and Intervention Across the Whole Spectrum of Allen Test Results," Journal of the American College of Cardiology, vol. 63, no. 18, pp. 1833-1841, May 2014, doi: 10.1016/j.jacc.2013.12.043.

[68] O. F. Bertrand, P. C. Carey, and I. C. Gilchrist, "Allen or No Allen," Journal of the American College of Cardiology, vol. 63, no. 18, pp. 1842-1844, May 2014, doi: 10.1016/j.jacc.2014.01.048.

[69] C. Bonnett, N. Becker, B. Hann, A. Haynes, and J. Tremmel, "Preventing Radial Artery Occlusion by Using Reverse Barbeau Assessment: Bringing Evidence-Based Practice to the Bedside," Critical Care Nurse, vol. 35, no. 4, pp. 77-82, August 2015, doi: 10.4037/ccn2015428.

[70] A. Mohamed Zarea, N. Taha Ahmed, and S. Elsayed Abdelmotalb Elsaman, "Comparison between modified Allen's test and Barbeau test for the assessment of hands' collateral circulation before arterial puncture among critically ill patients," International Journal of Africa Nursing Sciences, vol. 15, p. 100338, 2021, doi: 10.1016/j.ijans.2021.100338.

[71] G. A. Sgueglia, A. Di Giorgio, A. Gaspardone, and A. Babunashvili, "Anatomic Basis and Physiological Rationale of Distal Radial Artery Access for Percutaneous Coronary and Endovascular Procedures," JACC: Cardiovascular Interventions, vol. 11, no. 20, pp. 2113-2119, Oct. 2018, doi: 10.1016/j.jcin.2018.04.045.

[72] P. O. Lim and Z. Elghamry, "Heparin-free distal radial artery approach to cardiac catheterization and the small radial recurrent artery," Br J Cardiol, 2021, doi: 10.5837/bjc.2021.039.

[73]A. Hadjivassiliou, F. Kiemeneij, S. Nathan, and D. Klass, "Ultrasound-guided access to the distal radial artery at the anatomical snuffbox for catheter-based vascular interventions: a technical guide," EuroIntervention, vol. 16, no. 16, pp. 1342-1348, March 2021, doi: 10.4244/EIJ- D-19-00555.

[74]A. Achim et al, "The Role of Ultrasound in Accessing the Distal Radial Artery at the Anatomical Snuffbox for Cardiovascular Interventions," Life, vol. 13, no. 1, p. 25, Dec. 2022, doi: 10.3390/life13010025.

[75]S. Mori et al, "A Comparative Analysis between Ultrasound-Guided and Conventional Distal Transradial Access for Coronary Angiography and Intervention," Journal of Interventional Cardiology, vol. 2020, pp. 1-8, Sept. 2020, doi: 10.1155/2020/7342732.

[76]Sgueglia GA, Hassan A, Harb S, Ford TJ, Koliastasis L, Milkas A, Zappi DM, Navarro Lecaro A, Ionescu E, Rankin S, Said CF, Kuiper B, Kiemeneij F, International Hand Function Study Following Distal Radial Access: The RATATOUILLE Study, JACC Cardiovasc Interv, no 27;15(12):1205-1215, June 2022, doi: 10.1016/j.jcin.2022.04.023.

[77]A. Achim et al, "Distal Radial Artery Access for Recanalization of Radial Artery Occlusion and Repeat Intervention: A Single Center Experience," JCM, vol. 11, no. 23, p. 6916, Nov. 2022, doi: 10.3390/jcm11236916.

[78]G. L. Gasparini, R. Garbo, A. Gagnor, J. Oreglia, and P. Mazzarotto, "First prospective multicentre experience with left distal transradial approach for coronary chronic total occlusion interventions using a 7 Fr Glidesheath Slender," EuroIntervention, vol. 15, no. 1, pp. 126-128, May 2019, doi: 10.4244/EIJ-D-18-00648.

[79]J. W. Roh et al, "The learning curve of the distal radial access for coronary intervention", Sci Rep, vol. 11, no. 1, p. 13217, June 2021, doi: 10.1038/s41598-021-92742-7.

[80]K. M. Al-Azizi et al, "The Left Distal Transradial Artery Access for Coronary Angiography and Intervention: A US Experience," Cardiovascular Revascularization Medicine, vol. 20, no. 9, pp. 786-789, Sept. 2019, doi: 10.1016/j.carrev.2018.10.023.

[81]M. A. Sadaka, W. Etman, W. Ahmed, S. Kandil, and S. Eltahan, "Incidence and predictors of radial artery occlusion after transradial coronary catheterization," Egypt Heart J, vol. 71, no. 1, p. 12, Dec. 2019, doi: 10.1186/s43044-019-0008-0.

[82]T. Wakeyama et al, "Distal radial arterial hypertrophy after transradial intervention: A serial intravascular ultrasound study," Journal of Cardiology, vol. 72, no. 6, pp. 501-505, Dec. 2018, doi: 10.1016/j.jjcc.2018.05.008.

[83]D. Horák, I. Bernat, Š. Jirouš, D. Slezák, and R. Rokyta, "Distal radial access and postprocedural ultrasound evaluation of proximal and distal radial artery," Cardiovasc Interv and Ther, vol. 37, no. 4, pp. 710-716, Oct. 2022, doi: 10.1007/s12928-022-00857-z.

[84]Flores EA, "Making the right move: use of the distal radial artery access in the hand for coronary angiography and percutaneous coronary interventions," Cath Lab Digest, pp. 16-25, 12 2018, [Online]. Available from: www.cathlabdigest.com.

[85] J.-W. Lee, S. W. Park, J.-W. Son, S.-G. Ahn, and S.-H. Lee, "Real-world experience of the left distal transradial approach for coronary angiography and percutaneous coronary intervention: a prospective observational study (LeDRA)," EuroIntervention, vol. 14, no. 9, pp. e995-e1003, Oct. 2018, doi: 10.4244/EIJ-D-18-00635.

[86] S. P. Prejean, G. Von Mering, and M. Ahmed, "Successful Treatment of Pseudoaneurysm Following Left Distal Transradial Cardiac Catheterization With Compression Device," Journal for Vascular Ultrasound, vol. 43, no. 2, pp. 81-85, June 2019, doi: 10.1177/1544316719844061.

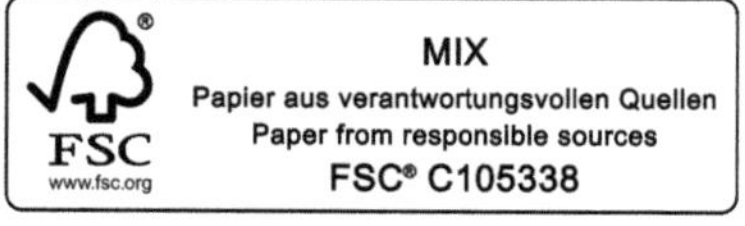

Printed by Books on Demand GmbH, Norderstedt / Germany